PSYCHOSOMATIC MEDICINE

Its Principles and Applications

BY

FRANZ ALEXANDER, M.D.

DIRECTOR, CHICAGO INSTITUTE FOR PSYCHOANALYSIS
CLINICAL PROFESSOR OF PSYCHIATRY, UNIVERSITY OF ILLINOIS

WITH A CHAPTER ON

*The Functions of the Sexual Apparatus
and Their Disturbances*

By THERESE BENEDEK, M.D.
MEMBER OF STAFF, CHICAGO INSTITUTE FOR PSYCHOANALYSIS

WITH A FOREWORD TO THE 1987 EDITION

By GEORGE H. POLLOCK, M.D., PH.D.
PRESIDENT, INSTITUTE FOR PSYCHOANALYSIS, CHICAGO

W · W · NORTON & COMPANY · NEW YORK · LONDON

TO MY COLLABORATORS IN THE
INSTITUTE OF PSYCHOANALYSIS, CHICAGO

Copyright © 1987, 1950 by W. W. Norton & Company, Inc.

Published simultaneously in Canada by Penguin Books Canada Ltd.
2801 John Street, Markham, Ontario L3R 1B4.

Printed in the United States of America.

Library of Congress Cataloging-in-Publication Data

Alexander, Franz, 1891–
    Psychosomatic medicine.

    Bibliography: p.
    Includes indexes.
    1. Medicine, Psychosomatic.   I. Benedek, Therese,
1892-   . II. Title. [DNLM: 1. Psychosomatic
Medicine.   WM 90 A375p]
RC49.A4   1987   616.08   86-31130

ISBN 0-393-70036-4

W. W. Norton & Company, Inc., 500 Fifth Avenue, New York, NY 10110

W. W. Norton & Company Ltd., 37 Great Russell Street, London WC1B 3NU

1 2 3 4 5 6 7 8 9 0

A NORTON PROFESSIONAL BOOK

Foreword to the 1987 Edition

GEORGE POLLOCK, M.D.

THE PIONEERING and exciting contributions of Franz Alexander to many areas of psychiatry, psychoanalysis, and medicine are well-known and acknowledged worldwide. Some of his ideas are still pivotal to our understanding of human psychology, and some are now once again coming to the fore in our clinical and theoretical considerations, forming the foundation for those who succeeded him and who are investigating new areas.

As reflected in this volume, one of Alexander's central research areas was mind-body interrelationships. This work rested on his clinical experiences of offering psychoanalytic treatment to patients with various physiological diseases, e.g., duodenal ulcer, ulcerative colitis, bronchial asthma, neurodermatitis, essential hypertension, rheumatoid arthritis, and thyrotoxicosis. Later many of Alexander's colleagues at the Chicago Institute for Psychoanalysis participated in these clinical studies. The result was a formal study of psychosomatic specificity (Alexander, French, and Pollock, 1968). This study confirmed Alexander's hypothesis about specificity and some of the formulations of the seven diseases that were investigated, and we can now extend the findings of his work and the specificity group into areas that heretofore were unexplored.

3

Alexander's writings on clinical and theoretical aspects of psychosomatic interrelationships are still utilized by students, teachers, researchers, and theoreticians of many disciplines. In particular, his early findings have inspired the resurgence of research into the relationship of brain-body-mind, affect-cognition-motivation, as new techniques have extended our understanding of healthy and pathological behavior.

Alexander's father was the professor of philosophy at the University of Budapest. He grew up in a household of scholarship, ideas, and intellectual stimulation. The effects of this childhood and his relationship with his father, as well as those with other stimulating figures, are seen in Alexander's writings. He was the philosopher, the seeker of universals, the explorer of ideas. At times he may have been wrong, but he learned from his errors and corrected his assumptions and misunderstandings. I saw this firsthand in our specificity prediction research. He had a facile mind, intuitive appreciation of patients' communications, and yet the impatience of a restless intellectual.

In Part One of this volume we can still detect the freshness of Alexander's thoughts in chapters dealing with historical, philosophical, nosological, etiological, methodological, and conceptual aspects of psychosomatic medicine—this despite the fact that this volume was first published in 1950. In Part Two Alexander included a chapter on sexuality and its dysfunctions, written by his long-time associate, Therese Benedek. Alexander had brought Benedek to the Chicago Institute for Psychoanalysis and encouraged her research studies, especially those dealing with sexuality. Her study of the female sexual cycle (conducted in collaboration with B. Rubenstein) is a classic (Benedek and Rubenstein, 1942) and in some ways served as a model for the later psychosomatic specificity predictive study noted above.

Alexander's final chapter on therapy is sketchy, general, and somewhat dated, but it represents his point of view when he wrote *Psychosomatic Medicine*. In this final chapter Alexander states that "Progress in modern medicine consists specifically in the co-operation of the psychiatric and non-psychiatric specialists both in diagnosis and in treatment" (p. 264). He goes on to point out that patients require "general medical care, dietary management, and pharmacological treatment" (p. 264). This is very much in line with current thinking about combining psychotherapy with pharmacotherapy. Alexander did not spell this out, as the various pharmacologic agents available at the time that he wrote this volume were somewhat limited, but one can see retrospectively how he was moving in a direction which now allows this type of combinatorial work where indicated. The combined use of pharmacological agents and dynamic psychotherapy is only now being widely accepted. It is likely that this therapeutic modality would have been acceptable to Alexander.

Alexander was cognizant of the emerging field of stress research and its relationship to neural and hormonal studies. Had he the opportunity to explore the current exciting advances in psychoneuroimmunology, cellular aspects of memory and learning, and findings that relate endorphins to many psychological processes, and the newer nosologies of DSM-III, he probably would have modified his theories, where such change was indicated.

The specificity hypothesis presented in *Psychosomatic Medicine* is still with us, with some elaborations, e.g., the idea of combinatorial specificity (Pollock, 1981) and the suggestion that there may be two or more diseases present at the same time in the same individual, each requiring different therapeutic approaches (Pollock, 1986). Research on the stress-strain disorders has expanded the list of diseases Alexander and his colleagues studied in their initial clinical and research investigations. Today we would include such entities as coronary heart disease, eating disorders, and diabetes. Newer epidemiologic and genetic research, gender differences, and age differences are but a few additional considerations that Alexander might have pursued.

This volume has served at least two generations of psychiatrists, psychoanalysts, psychologists, social workers, nurses, students, teachers, researchers, and practitioners in other medical disciplines who encounter the "psychosomatic" patient. I welcome its reissue as a worthy tribute to a pioneer whose work has been a stimulus to many who followed him.

REFERENCES

Alexander, Franz, French, Thomas M., and Pollock, George H. (1968), *Psychosomatic Specificity: Experimental Study and Results*. Chicago: University of Chicago Press.

Benedek, Therese, and Rubenstein, Boris B. (1942), *The Sexual Cycle in Women: The Relation Between Ovarian Function and Psychodynamic Processes*. Washington, D.C.: National Research Council.

Pollock, George H. (1981), Combinatorial specificity and the complemental series. *The Annual of Psychoanalysis*, IX:161–171. Madison, Connecticut: International Universities Press.

Pollock, George H. (1986), Do multiple diseases exist simultaneously? *The Annual of Psychoanalysis*, XIV:143–146. Madison, Connecticut: International Universities Press.

Contents

7

Contents

Foreword

THIS BOOK, an outgrowth of an earlier publication, *The Medical Value of Psychoanalysis,* has two objectives. It attempts to describe the basic concepts on which the psychosomatic approach in medicine is founded and to present the existing knowledge concerning the influence of psychological factors upon the functions of the body and their disturbances. It does not contain an exhaustive review of the many isolated incidental observations published in medical literature concerning emotional influences upon disease; it presents only the results of systematic investigations.

The author's conviction is that progress in this field requires the acceptance of a basic postulate: that the psychological factors influencing physiological processes must be subjected to the same detailed and careful scrutiny as is customary in the study of physiological processes. Reference to emotions in such general terms as anxiety, tension, emotional imbalance is outdated. The actual psychological content of an emotion must be studied with the most advanced methods of dynamic psychology and correlated with bodily responses. Only such studies are included in this book as are carried out in accordance with this methodological principle.

Another postulate which characterizes this writing is that

psychological processes are fundamentally not different from other processes which take place in the organism. They are at the same time physiological processes and differ from other body processes only in that they are perceived subjectively and can be communicated verbally to others. They can therefore be studied by psychological methods. Every bodily process is directly or indirectly influenced by psychological stimuli because the whole organism constitutes a unit with all of its parts interconnected. The psychosomatic approach therefore can be applied to every phenomenon which takes place in the living organism. This universality of application justifies one's speaking of a psychosomatic era in medicine. At present there can be no doubt that the psychosomatic point of view offers a new approach to the understanding of the organism as an integrated mechanism. Therapeutic possibilities are established in many chronic diseases and encourage the hope for further application in the future.

Chicago, December, 1949

Acknowledgments

THE PSYCHOSOMATIC approach is a multidiscipline procedure in which psychiatrists collaborate with experts in the different branches of medicine. This book is the result of seventeen years' collaboration with my colleagues in the Chicago Institute for Psychoanalysis and other medical specialists.

I wish to thank Dr. I. Arthur Mirsky for his assistance in evaluating some of the physiological data, in particular in the sections on hormonal mechanisms, anorexia nervosa, hypertension, thyrotoxicosis, and diabetes mellitus, and the preparation of illustrations, and Miss Helen Ross, Drs. Thomas Szasz and George Ham, who have read the manuscript and made valuable suggestions. The chapter on thyrotoxicosis is based on investigative work which I carried out in collaboration with Dr. George Ham and Dr. Hugh Carmichael, the results of which will be published in *The Journal of Psychosomatic Medicine*.

Some chapters of the manuscript are based on previously published articles. I wish to thank Dr. Carl A. L. Binger and Paul B. Hoeber, Inc. for their permission to reprint parts of articles previously published in *Psychosomatic Medicine* (F. Alexander: "Psychological Aspects of Medicine," "Emotional Factors in Essential Hypertension," "Psychoanalytic Study of a

Case of Essential Hypertension," "Treatment of a Case of Peptic Ulcer and Personality Disorder"; F. Alexander and S. A. Portis: "A Psychosomatic Study of Hypoglycaemic Fatigue"), Dr. Sidney Portis for allowing me to reprint sections of my chapter published in *Diseases of the Digestive System*, the National Safety Council of Chicago for permission to reprint my article published in *Current Topics in Home Safety*, and Dr. Iago Galdston and Henry H. Wiggins for their permission to reprint parts of my article, "Present Trends in Psychiatry and the Future Outlook," published in *Modern Attitudes in Psychiatry*, Columbia University Press, which served as a basis for parts of the introduction and certain sections in the first five chapters.

Part One

General Principles

Chapter I

Introduction

ONCE AGAIN, the patient as a human being with worries, fears, hopes, and despairs, as an indivisible whole and not merely the bearer of organs—of a diseased liver or stomach—is becoming the legitimate object of medical interest. In the last two decades increasing attention has been paid to the causative role of emotional factors in disease. A growing psychological orientation manifests itself among physicians. Some sound and conservative clinicians deem this a threat to the foundations of medicine so arduously acquired, and authoritative voices warn the profession that this new "psychologism" is incompatible with medicine as a natural science. They would prefer that medical psychology remain restricted to the field of medical art, to tact and intuition in handling the patient, as distinct from the scientific procedure of therapy proper based on physics, chemistry, anatomy, and physiology.

From a historical perspective, however, this psychological interest is nothing more than a revival of old pre-scientific views in a new and scientific form. The care of the suffering man has not always been divided between the priest and the physician. Once the healing functions, mental and physical, were united in one hand. Whatever the explanation of the healing power of the medicine man or of the evangelist or of the holy water of Lourdes, there is little doubt that these agents often achieved a spectacular curative effect upon the sick, in certain respects even more dramatic than many of our drugs which we can analyze chemically and the pharmacological effects of which we know with great precision. This psychological aspect of medicine survived only in a rudimentary form as the art of medicine and the bedside manner, carefully separated from the scientific aspect of therapy, and thought of chiefly as the suggestive, reassuring influence of the physician upon his patient.

Modern scientific medical psychology is but an attempt to place medical art, the psychological effect of the physician upon the patient, on a scientific basis and to make it an integral part of therapy. There is little doubt that much of the therapeutic success of the healing profession, of the medicine man and of the priest as well as of the modern practitioner, has been due to the undefined emotional rapport between physician and patient. This psychological function of the physician, however, was largely disregarded in the last century, when medicine became a genuine natural science based on the application of the principles of physics and chemistry to the living organism. The fundamental philosophical postulate of modern medicine is that the body and its functions can be understood in terms of physical chemistry that living organisms are physicochemical machines and the ideal of the physician is to become an engineer of the body. The recognition of psychological forces, a psychological approach to the problems of life and disease, appears to some as a relapse to the ignorance of the dark ages when disease was considered as the work of an evil spirit and therapy was exorcism, the expelling of the demon from the diseased body. It was natural that the new medicine based on laboratory experiments should have jealously defended its newly acquired scientific halo against such antiquated mystical concepts as those of psychology. Medicine, this newcomer among the natural sciences, in many respects assumed the attitude typical of the newcomer who wants to make one forget his lowly origin and becomes more intolerant, exclusive, and conservative than the genuine aristocrat. Medicine became intolerant toward everything which was reminiscent of its spiritual and mystical past, at a time when its older brother, physics, the aristocrat of the natural sciences, was undergoing the most profound revision of its fundamental concepts, questioning even the shibboleth of science, the general validity of determinism.

These remarks are not intended to minimize the accomplishments of the laboratory period in medicine, the most brilliant phase of its history. The physicochemical orientation characterized by the precise study of fine details is responsible for the great progress of medicine exemplified by modern bacteriology, surgery, and pharmacology. It is one of the paradoxes of historical development that the greater the scientific merits of a method or principle, the greater will be its effect in retarding subsequent developments. The inertia of the human mind makes it stick to ideas and methods which have proved of value in the past even though their usefulness has served its turn. Many examples may be found in the development of the exact sciences such as physics. Einstein maintained that Aristotle's ideas of motion retarded the development of mechanics for two thousand years (76). Progress in every field requires a reorientation with the introduction of new principles. Although these new principles may actually not be contradictory to the old ones, they are often rejected or accepted only after much struggle for recognition.

The scientist in this respect is just as narrow-minded as the man in the street. The same physicochemical orientation to which medicine owes its greatest accomplishments has become on account of its one-sidedness an obstacle to further development. The laboratory era of medicine was characterized by its analytic attitude. Typical of this period was a specialized interest in detailed mechanisms, in the understanding of partial processes. The discovery of finer methods of observation, especially through the microscope, disclosed a new microcosm by giving an unprecedented insight into the minute parts of the body. In the study of the causes of diseases, the principal aim thus became the localization of the pathological processes. In ancient medicine the humoral theory prevailed, claiming the fluids of the body to be the carriers of disease. The gradual development of methods of autopsy during the Renaissance made possible a precise study of the details of the human organism and thus led to more realistic but at the same time more localistic etiological concepts. Morgagni, in the middle of the eighteenth century, claimed that the seat of various diseases was in particular organs such as the heart, the kidney, the liver, etc. With the introduction of the microscope the localization of disease became even more confined: the cell became the seat of the disease. It was Virchow, to whom pathology owes so much, who declared that there are no general diseases, only diseases of organs and of cells. His great achievements in pathology and his authority established a dogma in cellular pathology, which has influenced medical thinking up to the present day. Virchow's influence upon etiological thought is the classical example of the historical paradox that the greatest accomplishments of the past become the greatest obstacles to further development. The observation of histological changes in diseased organs made possible by the microscope and by the refined techniques of staining tissues determined the pattern for etiological thought. Search for the cause of disease long remained limited to the search for local morphological changes in tissues. The concept that such local anatomical changes themselves may result from more general disturbances which develop in consequence of faulty function, excessive stress, or even emotional factors remained to be discovered much later. The less particularistic humoral theory, which became discredited when Virchow successfully defeated its last repre-

sentative, Rokitansky, had to wait for its revival in the form
of modern endocrinology.

Few have understood the essence of this phase of medical
development better than Stefan Zweig, a layman. In his book,
Mental Healers, he says,[1]

> Disease meant now no longer what happens to the whole man
> but what happens to his organs. . . . And so the natural and
> original mission of the physician, the approach to disease as a
> whole changes into the smaller task of localizing the ailment and
> identifying it and ascribing it to an already specified group of
> diseases. . . . This unavoidable objectification and technical-
> ization of therapy in the nineteenth century came to an extreme
> excess because between the physician and the patient became
> interpolated a third entirely mechanical thing, the apparatus.
> The penetrating, creative synthesizing grasp of the born physi-
> cian became less and less necessary for diagnosis. . . .

Not less impressive is the statement of Alan Gregg, a hu-
manitarian who views the past and future of medicine in a
broad perspective: [2]

> The totality that is a human being has been divided for study
> into parts and systems; one cannot decry the method but one
> is not obliged to remain satisfied with its results alone. What
> brings and keeps our several organs and numerous functions in
> harmony and federation? And what has medicine to say of the
> facile separation of "mind" from "body"? What makes an in-
> dividual what the word implies—not divided? The need for
> more knowledge here is of an excruciating obviousness. But
> more than mere need there is a foreshadowing of changes to
> come. Psychiatry is astir, neurophysiology is crescent, neuro-
> surgery flourishes, and a star still hangs over the cradle of en-
> docrinology. . . . Contributions from other fields are to seek
> from psychology, cultural anthropology, sociology and philos-
> ophy as well as from chemistry and physics and internal medi-
> cine to resolve the dichotomy of mind and body left us by
> Descartes.

[1] Stefan Zweig: *Die Heilung durch den Geist* (Mental Healers). Leipzig,
Insel-Verlag, 1931.
[2] Alan Gregg: "The Future of Medicine," *Harvard Medical Alumni Bulletin,*
Cambridge, October 1936.

Thus modern clinical medicine was divided into two heterogeneous portions, one, considered the more advanced and scientific, which includes all disturbances that can be explained in terms of physiology and general pathology (for example, organic heart defects, diabetes, infectious disease, etc.), and the other, considered less scientific, which includes a great conglomeration of ailments of obscure, frequently psychic origin. Characteristic of this dual attitude—a typical manifestation of the inertia of the human mind—is the tendency to force more and more diseases into the etiological scheme of infection, where pathogenic cause and pathological effect appear to have a comparatively simple relationship to each other. When the infectious or other organic explanation fails, the modern clinician is only too ready to console himself with the hope that sometime in the future, after more details of the organic processes are known, the psychic factor, unwillingly admitted, will eventually be eliminated. And yet, gradually, more and more clinicians with a broader perspective have come to recognize that even in physiologically well-understood disturbances such as diabetes or essential hypertension only the last links in the causal chain are known and the primary etiological factors still remain in darkness. In these, as in other chronic conditions, accumulated observations seem to point to "central" factors, the expression "central" being obviously a mere euphemism for "psychogenic."

This state of affairs easily explains the peculiar discrepancy between the official-theoretical and the factual-practical attitude of the physician in his practice. In his scientific contributions, in his addresses to medical groups, he will stress the need for knowing more and more details about the underlying physiological and pathological processes, and he will refuse to believe seriously in psychogenic etiology; in his private practice, however, he will without hesitation advise his patient suffering from essential hypertension to try to relax, take life less seriously, and avoid overwork, and he will try to convince his patient that his overactive, overambitious attitude in life is the real source of his high blood pressure. This "dual personality" of the modern clinician reveals more clearly than anything else the weak spot in present-day medicine. Within the medical community, the practitioner can afford to assume a "scientific" attitude which is essentially only a dogmatic antipsychological attitude. Because he does not know exactly how this psychic element works, because it is so contradictory to everything he has learned during his medical training, and because the recognition of the psychic factor seemingly disrupts the consistency of the physicochemical theory of life, such a practitioner tries to disregard the psychic factor as much as possible. As a physician, however, he cannot entirely disregard it. Confronted with his patients, his therapeutic conscience forces him to pay primary attention to this detested factor, the importance of which he instinctively senses. He must deal with it, but in doing so he excuses himself with the phrase that medical healing is not only a science but an art as well. He is unaware that what he refers to as medical art is nothing but the deeper, intuitive—i.e., unverbalized—knowledge which he has obtained during the long years of his clinical experience. The significance of psychiatry, particularly of the psychoanalytic method, for the development of medicine lies in the fact that it supplies an efficient technique for the study of the psychological factors in disease.

Chapter II

The Role of Modern Psychiatry in the Development of Medicine

IT WAS reserved for psychiatry, the most neglected and least developed specialty in medicine, to introduce a new synthetic approach into medicine. During the greater portion of the laboratory period of medicine, psychiatry remained a rather isolated domain with little contact with the other specialties. Psychiatry was concerned with the mentally diseased, a field in which the commonly accepted methods of healing were least effective. The symptomatology of mental disturbances differed unpleasantly from the disorders of the body. Psychiatry dealt with delusions, hallucinations, and the disturbances of emotional life, symptoms which could not be described in the usual terms of medicine. Inflammation can be described in such physical terms as swelling, increased temperature, and definite microscopic changes in the cells. Tuberculosis is diagnosed by definite changes in the afflicted tissues and by the presence of well-defined microorganisms. Pathological mental functions, however, had to be described in psychological terms, and consequently etiological understanding based on current medical concepts was hardly applicable to mental disturbances. This difference separated psychiatry from the rest of medicine. In their effort to bridge this gap, some psychiatrists tried to explain mental symptoms by assuming without sufficient foundation hypothetical disturbances of body functions, a trend which to some degree exists even today.

A more scientific approach to this impasse was the effort to make the psychological description of mental diseases more precise and systematic. If the psychiatrist was unable to explain disturbed mental symptoms by the methods of other medical disciplines, he at least tried to present his observations in a detailed and systematic fashion. This trend characterized the period of descriptive psychiatry under the leadership of men like Kahlbaum, Wernicke, Babinski, and finally Kraepelin, who gave modern psychiatry its first comprehensive and reliable descriptive system of mental disease entities.

At the same time the attempt to apply to psychiatry the principles of localization of disease, as expounded by Morgagni and Virchow, was stubbornly pursued by the leading medical minds of the nineteenth century. That the brain is the seat of psychological functions was known, in a general fashion at least, to the physicians of ancient Greece. With increased knowledge of brain physiology and anatomy it became possible to localize various perceptive and motor systems in the different cortical and subcortical areas of the brain. This, together with advancing histological procedures, gave rise to the hope that the understanding of mental functions and diseases might come from the knowledge of the complex cellular structure of the brain (cytoarchitectonics). The studies of Cajal, Golgi, Nissl, Alzheimer, Apathy, von Lenhossek, and many others which yielded extremely refined and detailed information concerning the histological structure of the brain are illustrative. These studies were characterized by their preponderantly descriptive nature, the functional significance of anatomical structures, particularly of the higher brain centers, remaining relatively unknown. In no other medical discipline was there such a great dichotomy between morphological and functional knowledge as in the field concerned with the study of the brain. Where, in the brain, thought processes and emotions take place, and how memory, volition, and reasoning are related to brain structure—all this was almost completely unexplored and remains even at the present time but little understood.

For such reasons many of the great psychiatrists of that era were primarily brain anatomists and were clinicians only secondarily. Their scientific and medical activity was characterized by the frustrating feeling that they could not unify their clinical observations with their knowledge of the anatomy and physiology of the brain. Some of them tried to bridge this gap by speculations concerning the psychological significance of brain structure, speculations to which the German physiologist, Max Verworn, referred as "brain mythology." The dichotomy between morphological and physiological knowledge of the brain is well illustrated by the remark of a physiologist who, after listening to an elaborate presentation of a histological paper by Karl Schaffer, the renowned brain anatomist and psychiatrist, said: "You brain anatomists remind me of the mailman who knows people's names and addresses, but has no idea what these people do."

At the turn of the century, this gap between anatomical and functional knowledge characterized the state of affairs in psychiatry. On the one hand stood the well-developed science of neuroanatomy and pathology, and on the other a reliable description of mental illnesses—each isolated from the other. A different state of affairs existed, however, so far as a purely "organic" understanding of the nervous system was concerned. Neurology, the sister branch of psychiatry, succeeded in unifying anatomical knowledge with the function of the organs. Localization of the co-ordination of voluntary and reflex motions had been carefully worked out. Disturbances of such highly co-ordinated movements as speech, grabbing, and walking could often be correlated either with damage to those parts of the nervous system in which the co-ordination of these innervations lies, or with damage to the peripheral nervous connections between the central co-ordinating parts of the nervous system and the disturbed organs of motility. In this manner neurology applied the principle of Morgagni and Virchow and became a respected, precise medical discipline, while psychiatry remained an obscure field.

At the same time, the vision of the student of neuro-anatomy of constructing a bridge between brain and mind, between psychiatry and brain anatomy and physiology, remained a utopia and continues to remain so to the present day.

The principle of Virchow has not proved so effective in the field of mental diseases as in other departments of medicine. The common major disturbances of the personality—the schizophrenic and manic-depressive psychoses—which had been described by Kahlbaum, Kraepelin, Bleuler, and other great clinicians could not be identified with the help of the microscope. Careful histological studies of the brain of deceased psychotics did not reveal any significant microscopic changes. The medical man was thus confronted with a puzzle. Why did the brain of a patient whose external behavior and emotional reactions differed so conspicuously from those of the healthy person not reveal any consistent histological deviations even under the most exacting scrutiny? The same question arose in respect to many other psychiatric conditions, such as the psychoneuroses and the behavior disorders. A first ray of hope of connecting the knowledge of brain structure and mental disturbances appeared when it was discovered that general paralysis, long suspected to be caused by syphilis, could be traced to tissue damage in the central nervous system. When Noguchi and Moore finally proved beyond doubt the syphilitic origin of general paralysis, new hope was felt that psychiatry would advance eventually into the ranks of the other medical specialties. Although the existence of structural changes of brain tissue in senile dementia and in Alzheimer's disease had been known for many years, Noguchi's discovery of the microorganism Treponema pallidum in the brain of the general paretic opened the way for the first time to an etiologically oriented therapy.

Etiology has a generally accepted classical pattern: the disease syndrome is due to the faulty functioning of some organ, which in turn is the result of a damage to cellular structures which can be recognized microscopically. The damage is attributed to various causes, the most important being infection—i.e., the invasion of an organ by microorganisms—as in tuberculosis, the action of chemical agents as in poisoning, and the effect of mechanical damage as in fractures or contusions. In addition, aging—the chronic deterioration of all living organisms—has also been recognized as an important causal factor of disease.

At the beginning of the century, these etiological views also prevailed in psychiatry. Concussions of the brain and hemorrhages causing pressure were examples of the mechanical causation of disturbed mental function; alcoholism and other toxic psychoses exemplified the chemical etiology; and senile dementia, a well-defined condition based on the progressive degeneration of brain tissue, was a result of aging. Finally, when in 1913 Noguchi announced his discovery, the syphilitic conditions of the nervous system, particularly general paralysis characterized by profound changes in the personality, could serve as the counterpart of the bacterial invasions of other organs, such as tuberculosis of the lungs.

Now the psychiatrist could raise his head; he could finally approach his patient with laboratory methods of diagnosis and treatment. Before Ehrlich's chemotherapy of post-syphilitic diseases, the role of the psychiatrist consisted in merely custodial care and, at the most, careful observation of the patient. Whatever therapy had existed was either based on magic, as in the exorcism of evil spirits of the prescientific era, or was completely ineffective, such as the electro- and hydrotherapy so popular at the end of the last and the beginning of this century. Ehrlich's discovery of salvarsan contributed immensely to the prestige of psychiatry. As a real causal therapy it satisfied all the demands of modern medical philosophy. It was directed toward the elimination of the established specific cause of the disease, a pathogenic microorganism. It followed the method of applying a powerful chemical substance designed to leave the organism unharmed and to exterminate the pathogenic agent. Under the influence of this discovery, hopes ran high that soon the whole field of psychiatry would yield to methods used in other branches of medical research and therapy. (Therapeutic results with chemotherapy of general paralysis have turned out to be much less satisfactory than was expected at the beginning. This therapy was later supplanted by the more effective fever treatment and still later by penicillin.)

Other impressive discoveries contributed to the hopeful outlook. The explanation of the symptoms of mental retardation in myxedema as resulting from a decreased function of the thyroid gland, and the remarkable cure by Horsley through transplantation of the thyroid gland (later supplanted by oral medication of thyroid extract) is another classic example of the causal organic treatment of a psychiatric condition.

In hyperthyroidism too the mental symptoms could be influenced by chemical and surgical methods. These two diseases showed beyond doubt that the endocrine glands have a definite influence upon mental processes. It was therefore not unreasonable to hope that with the advancement of biochemistry, particularly with the intimate knowledge of the complicated interplay of the endocrine glands, the physiological causes of psychoses and psychoneuroses would be understood and made accessible to effective therapy.

Except for the existence of the important group of schizophrenic disturbances, in 'which a profound disintegration of the personality occurs without any discernible organic change, and of the even larger group of psychoneuroses, psychiatry in the second decade of this century might have become a branch of medicine like internal medicine, based on pathological anatomy and physiology, and using traditional methods of treatment. We shall see, however, that the development of psychiatry took a different course. Psychiatry did not become converted to an exclusively organic point of view. Rather, general medicine began to adopt an orientation which originated in psychiatry. This is called the psychosomatic point of view, and it introduced a new era of medicine: the psychosomatic era. How all this happened is of particular interest for the understanding of the present trend in medical evolution.

Chapter III

The Influence of Psychoanalysis upon the Development of Medicine

IN SPITE of sporadic successes, such as the explanation and treatment of general paralysis and myxedema by means of traditional methods of medicine, the majority of psychiatric conditions, the schizophrenic psychoses and the psychoneuroses, stubbornly resisted all efforts to bring them into the accepted framework. Major disturbances of the personality as well as the milder emotional disorders came to be regarded as "functional" diseases, in contrast to general paralysis or senile dementia, which are called "organic" because of the demonstrable structural changes in brain tissue. This terminological differentiation, however, did not alter the embarrassing fact that the disintegrations of psychic functions in schizophrenia resisted all types of therapy, such as pharmacological and surgical methods, and at the same time did not yield to any explanation along traditional lines. Yet the rapid progress in the application of laboratory methods in the rest of medicine was so promising that hope was not abandoned for a final understanding of all psychiatric disorders on an anatomical, physiological, and biochemical basis.

In all centers of medical research, histopathological, bacteriological, and biochemical attempts to solve the problem of schizophrenia and of other functional disturbances of the mind continued with unabated intensity into the last decade of the past century, when a completely novel method of investigation and therapy was introduced by Sigmund Freud. It is customary to attribute the origin of psychoanalysis to the French school, to the hypnosis research of Charcot, Bernheim, and Liébault. In his autobiographical writings, Freud traces the beginnings of his ideas to influences received during his studies in the Salpetrière with Charcot and later in Nancy with Bernheim and Liébault. From the point of view of biography, this is certainly a correct picture. From the point of view of the history of scientific thought, the beginning of the psychodynamic approach to mental disease must be credited to Freud himself.

As Galileo was the first to apply scientific reasoning to the phenomena of terrestrial motion, so Freud was the first to apply it in the study of human personality. Personality research or motivational psychology as a science begins with Freud. He was the first to adopt consistently the postulate of strict determinism of psychological processes and to establish the fundamental dynamic principle of psychological causality. After he discovered that a great part of human behavior is determined by unconscious motivations and after he developed a technique by which unconscious motivations can be made conscious, he was able to demonstrate for the first time the genesis of psychopathological processes. With the help of this new approach, the bizarre phenomena of psychotic and neurotic symptoms as well as seemingly senseless dreams could be understood as meaningful products of the mind. In the course of time, some details of his original views underwent modification, but most of his fundamental concepts have been validated by later observations. What is most permanent in his contribution is the method of observing human behavior and the type of reasoning he applied to its psychological understanding.

Historically viewed, the development of psychoanalysis can be considered as one of the first signs of a reaction against the one-sided analytical development of medicine in the second half of the nineteenth century, against the specialized interest in detailed mechanisms, against the neglect of the fundamental biological fact that the organism is one unit and the function of its parts can only be understood from the point of view of the whole system. The laboratory approach to the living organism had disclosed an incredible collection of more or less disconnected details, and this inevitably led to a loss of perspective. The view of the organism as a most ingenious mechanism in which every part co-operates for definite purposes had been either ignored or denounced as unsoundly teleological. It was claimed that the organism develops through certain natural causes but not for a certain purpose. A man-made machine, of course, could be understood on a teleological basis; the human mind created it for a certain definite purpose. But man was not created by a supreme intelligence—this was just the mythological concept from which modern biology fled, insisting that the animal body should be understood not on a teleological but on a causal and mechanistic basis.

As soon, however, as medicine, *nolens volens,* turned toward the problem of the diseased mind, this dogmatic attitude—at least in this field—had to be abandoned. In a study of personality, the fact that the organism is an intelligibly co-ordinated unit is so strikingly apparent that it cannot be overlooked. William White expressed this fact in simple terms: [1]

[1] William White: *The Meaning of Disease.* Baltimore, Williams & Wilkins, 1926.

The answer to the question: What is the function of the stomach?—is digestion, which is but a small part of the activity of the total organism and only indirectly, though of course importantly, related to many of its other functions. But if we undertake to answer the question, What is the man doing? we reply in terms of the total organism by saying, for example, that he is walking down the street or running a foot race or going to the theatre or studying medicine or what not. . . . If mind is the expression of a total reaction in distinction from a partial reaction, then every living organism must be credited with mental, that is, total types of response. . . . What we know as mind in all its present infinite complexity is the culmination of a type of response to the living organism that is historically as old as the bodily types of response with which we are more familiar. . . .

Personality can thus be defined as the expression of the unity of the organism. As a machine can only be understood from its function and purpose, the understanding of the synthetic unit which we call the body can only be fully understood from the point of view of the personality, the needs of which are served, in the last analysis, by all parts of the body in an intelligible co-ordination.

Psychiatry as the study of morbid personality was therefore to become the gateway for the introduction of the synthetic point of view into medicine. But psychiatry could accomplish this function only after it had discovered the study of personality as its main axis, and this was the accomplishment of Sigmund Freud. Psychoanalysis consists in the precise and detailed study of the development and functions of the personality. In spite of the fact that the term "psychoanalysis" contains the word "analysis," its historical significance consists not in its analytic but in its synthetic point of view.

Chapter IV

The Contributions of Gestalt Psychology, Neurology, and Endocrinology

PSYCHOANALYSIS, however, was not the only scientific movement toward synthesis. This trend was observable, at the turn of the century, in all fields of science. During the nineteenth century the development of scientific methods had resulted in the collection of data; discovery of new facts had become the highest goal. But the interpretation and correlation of these facts in the form of synthetic concepts had been looked upon with suspicion as unsound speculation or philosophy in contrast to science. As a reaction to this excessively analytic orientation, a strong desire for synthesis appeared as a general trend of the last decade of the century.

This new synthetic trend pervaded non-medical psychology. Here too the tradition of the nineteenth century had been the analytic approach. After the introduction into psychology of the experimental method by Fechner and Weber, psychological laboratories sprang up in which the human mind was dissected into its parts. There developed a psychology of vision, of hearing, of the tactile sense, of memory, of volition.

But the experimental psychologist never even tried to understand the interrelationships of all these different mental faculties and their integration into what we call the human personality. Köhler's, Wertheimer's and Koffka's Gestalt psychology can be regarded as a reaction against this particularistic analytic orientation. Probably the most important accomplishment of these Gestalt psychologists has been the clear formulation of the thesis that the whole is not the sum total of its parts but something different from them and that from the study of the parts alone the whole system never can be understood; that, in fact, just the opposite is true—the parts can be thoroughly understood only after the meaning of the whole has been discovered.

In medicine, a similar development has taken place. Advances in the field of neurology had paved the way for a more comprehensive understanding of the relationship between the different parts of the body. It became evident that all parts of the body are connected directly or indirectly with a central governing system and function under the control of this central organ. The voluntary muscles as well as the vegetative organs, the latter via the autonomic (vegetative) nervous system, are influenced by the highest centers of the nervous system. The unity of the organism is clearly expressed in the functions of the central nervous system, which regulates both the internal vegetative processes of the organism and also its external affairs, its relations to the environment. This central government is represented by the highest centers of the nervous system, the psychological aspects of which in human beings we call the personality. In fact, it is now obvious that physiological studies of the highest centers of the central nervous system and psychological studies of the personality deal with different aspects of one and the same thing. Whereas physiology approaches the functions of the central nervous system in terms of space and time, psychology approaches them in terms of various subjective phenomena which are *the subjective reflections of physiological processes.*

Another stimulus for the synthetic point of view came from the discovery of the ductless glands, a further step toward the understanding of the extremely complicated interrelationships between the different vegetative functions of the organism. The system of endocrine glands can be considered as a regulating system similar to that of the nervous system. Whereas the governing influence of the central nervous system is expressed through the conduction of regulating nervous impulses via the peripheral nerve pathways to the different parts of the body, the chemical regulation by the ductless glands takes place through the transportation of specific chemical substances by the blood stream.

It is now known that the rate of metabolism is primarily regulated by the product of the thyroid gland, that carbohydrate metabolism is regulated by the opposing influences of the internal secretion of the pancreas on the one hand and the hormones of the anterior pituitary and adrenal glands on the other, and that the master gland which co-ordinates the secretion of the peripheral endocrine glands is the anterior pituitary.

Recently, more and more evidence is emerging to indicate that most functions of the ductless glands are probably subject ultimately to the function of the highest centers of the brain, that is to say, to the psychic life.

These physiological discoveries gave us an insight into the mechanism of how the mind rules the body and how peripheral body functions in turn influence the central functions of the nervous system. The fact that the mind rules the body is, in spite of its neglect by biology and medicine, the most fundamental fact which we know about the process of life. This fact we observe continuously during all our life, from the moment when we awaken every morning. Our whole life consists in carrying out voluntary movements aimed at the realization of ideas and wishes, the satisfaction of subjective feelings such as thirst and hunger. The body, that complicated machine, carries out the most complex and refined motor activities under the influence of such psychological phenomena as ideas and wishes. The most specifically human of all bodily functions, speech, is but the expression of ideas through a refined musical instrument, the vocal apparatus. All our emotions we express through physiological processes: sorrow, by weeping; amusement, by laughter; and shame, by blushing. All emotions are accompanied by physiological changes: fear, by palpitation of the heart; anger, by increased heart activity, elevation of blood pressure, and changes in carbohydrate metabolism; despair, by a deep inspiration and expiration called sighing. All these physiological phenomena are the results of complex muscular interactions under the influence of nervous impulses, carried to the expressive muscles of the face and to the diaphragm in laughter, to the lacrimal glands in weeping, to the heart in fear, and to the adrenal glands and to the vascular system in rage. The nervous impulses arise in certain emotional situations which in turn originate from our interaction with other people. The originating psychological situations can be understood only in terms of psychology—as total responses of the organism to its environment.

Chapter V

Conversion Hysteria, Vegetative Neurosis, and Psychogenic Organic Disturbance

THE APPLICATION of these considerations to certain morbid processes of the body has gradually led to a new trend in medicine, to "psychosomatic medicine."

The psychosomatic point of view meant a new approach to the study of the causation of disease. As mentioned before, the fact that acute emotions have an influence on body functions belongs to everyday experience. Corresponding to every emotional situation there is a specific syndrome of physical changes, psychosomatic responses, such as laughter, weeping, blushing, changes in the heart rate, respiration, etc. However, since these psychomotor processes belong to our everyday life and have no ill effects, medicine has, until recently, paid little attention to a detailed investigation of them.[1] These changes in the body as reactions to acute emotions are of a passing nature. When the emotion disappears, the corresponding physiological process, weeping or laughter, heart

[1] One of the notable exceptions is Darwin (59).

palpitation or elevation of blood pressure, also disappears and the body returns to its equilibrium.

The psychoanalytic study of neurotic patients revealed, however, that under the influence of prolonged emotional disturbances, chronic disturbances of the body may develop. Such chronic bodily changes under the influence of emotion were first observed in hysterical patients. Freud introduced the concept of "conversion hysteria," in which bodily symptoms develop in response to chronic emotional conflicts. These changes were noted in the muscles controlled by the will and in sense perceptions. One of the most important discoveries of Freud was that when emotion cannot be expressed and relieved through normal channels by voluntary activity it may become the source of chronic psychic and physical disorders. Whenever emotions are repressed because of psychic conflicts—that is to say, excluded from consciousness and thus cut off from adequate discharge—they provide the source of chronic tension which is the cause of the hysterical symptoms.

From the physiological point of view, a hysterical conversion symptom is similar in nature to any usual voluntary innervation, expressive movement, or sensory perception. In hysteria, however, the motivating psychological impulse is unconscious. In attacking someone, or in going to a certain place, our arms and legs are put into motion under the influence of conscious motivations and goals. The so-called expressive movements such as laughter, weeping, grimacing, gesticulating, are based on similar physiological processes. In the latter, however, the innervations take place not under the influence of conscious goals but under the stimulus of an emotional tension which is discharged in a complex physiological pattern. In a conversion symptom like hysterical paralysis or contracture "the leap from the psychic to the somatic" is not different from the leap which takes place in any common motor innervation such as voluntary movements or laughter or weeping. Apart from the fact that the motivating psychological content is unconscious, the only difference is that hysterical conversion symptoms are to a high degree individual, sometimes unique creations of the patient, invented by him for the expression of his particular repressed psychological content. Expressive movements like laughter are in contrast standardized and universal (Darwin—59).

A fundamentally different group of psychogenic bodily disturbances is that involving the internal vegetative organs. Earlier psychoanalytic authors have repeatedly attempted to extend the original concept of hysterical conversion to all forms of psychogenic disturbances of the body, including those which occur in the visceral organs. According to such views an elevation of the blood pressure or a gastric hemorrhage has a symbolic meaning like any conversion symptom. No attention was paid to the fact that the vegetative organs are controlled by the autonomic nervous system, which is not in direct connection with ideational processes. Symbolic expression of psychological content is known only in the field of voluntary innervations such as speech, or expressive movements, such as facial grimacing, gesticulation, laughter, weeping, etc. Possibly blushing could be included in this group. It is most improbable, however, that internal organs such as the liver or the small arterioles of the kidney can symbolically express ideas. This does not mean that they cannot be influenced by emotional tensions, which can be conducted to any part of the body via cortico-thalamic and autonomic pathways. It is well established that emotional influences can stimulate or inhibit the function of any organ. After the emotional tension relaxes, the body functions return to their normal equilibrium. Whenever such emotional stimulation or inhibition of a vegetative function becomes chronic and excessive, we refer to it as an "organ neurosis." This term embraces the so-called "functional" disturbances of the vegetative organs, which are caused at least partially by nervous impulses the ultimate origins of which are emotional processes which take place somewhere in the cortical and subcortical areas of the brain.

The concept of functional disturbances came originally not from psychiatrists but from specialists in the field of internal diseases. At first the neurotic (or functional) disturbances of the stomach, the bowels, and the cardio-vascular system became known under the name of gastric, intestinal, or cardiac neuroses. The term "functional disturbance" refers to the fact that in such cases even the finest study of the tissues does not reveal any discernible morphological changes. The anatomical structure of the organ is not changed; only the coordination and the intensity of its functions are disturbed. Such disturbances are more readily reversible, and are considered less serious, than diseases in which the tissues show definite morphological alteration, which frequently designates irreversible damage.

We can now define the difference between conversion symptom and vegetative neurosis. A conversion symptom is a *symbolic* expression of an emotionally charged psychological content: it is an attempt to discharge the emotional tension. It takes place in the voluntary neuromuscular or sensory-perceptive systems whose original function is to express and relieve emotional tensions. A vegetative neurosis is not an attempt to express an emotion but is the physiological response of the vegetative organs to constant or to periodically returning emotional states. Elevation of blood pressure, for example, under the influence of rage does not relieve the rage but is a physiological component of the total phenomenon of rage. As will be shown later, it is an adaptation of the body to the state of the organism when it prepares to meet an emergency. Similarly, increased gastric secretion under the influence of emotional longing for food is not an expression or relief of these emotions; it is the adaptive preparation of the stomach for the incorporation of food.

The only similarity between hysterical conversion symptoms and vegetative responses to emotions lies in the fact that both are responses to psychological stimuli. They are basically different, however, in their psychodynamics and physiology.

With the recognition that in functional disturbances emotional factors are of causal significance, psychotherapy gained a legitimate entrance into medicine proper and could no longer be restricted exclusively to the field of psychiatry. The chronic emotional conflicts of the patient, the ultimate cause of the disturbance, had to be resolved by psychological treatment. Since these emotional conflicts arose in the patient's relationships with other human beings, the personality of the patient became the object of therapy. With this new emphasis, the emotional influence of the doctor upon the patient—medical art—found its place in scientific medicine. It could no longer be considered an appendage of therapy, a last artistic touch in therapeutic skill. In cases of organ neuroses the emotional influence of the physician upon the patient proved to be the main therapeutic factor.

The role of psychotherapy remained restricted, however, at this phase of development, to the functional cases generally considered as milder disturbances in contrast to the genuine organic disorders based on demonstrable tissue changes. In such organic disorders too, the emotional state of the patient had long been recognized as an important issue; yet a real causal connection between psychic factors and genuine organic disturbances had not been generally assumed.

Gradually, however, it became increasingly evident that nature does not know such strict distinctions as "functional" versus "organic." Clinicians began to suspect that functional disorders of long duration may gradually lead to serious organic disorders associated with morphological changes. A few instances of this kind have been known for a long time—for example, the fact that hyperactivity of the heart may lead to hypertrophy of the heart muscles or that hysterical paralysis of a limb may lead to certain degenerative changes in the muscles and joints because of inactivity. One had to reckon, therefore, with the possibility that a functional disturbance of long duration in any organ may lead finally to definite anatomical changes and to the clinical picture of severe organic illness. Intensive psychological and physiological studies of cases of peptic ulcer brought convincing evidence for the view that emotional conflicts of long duration may lead as a first step to a stomach neurosis which in time may result in an ulcer. There are also indications that emotional conflicts may cause continued fluctuations of blood pressure which in time overtax the vascular system. This functional phase of fluctuating blood pressure may in time cause organic vascular changes, and finally an irreversible malignant form of hypertension may ensue.

These observations have been crystallized in the concept of "psychogenic organic disorder." These disorders, according to this view, develop in two phases: first, the functional disturbance of a vegetative organ is caused by a chronic emotional disturbance; and second, the chronic functional disturbance gradually leads to tissue changes, and to an irreversible organic disease.

Chapter VI

Progress in Etiological Thought

FORMERLY every disturbed function was explained as the *result* of disturbed structure. Now another causal sequence has been established: disturbed function as the *cause* of altered structure. Although this etiological view is not entirely novel, many clinicians raised in the tradition of Virchow's principle and still under the impressive influence of the simple and experimentally validated etiological discoveries of bacteriology are disinclined to accept it without reservations. When a functional disorder is described as resulting from emotional conflict, the idea is usually accepted with some doubt by the traditional clinician and the hope is expressed that further, more precise histological studies will eventually disclose tissue changes responsible for the disease. He is inclined to fall back upon the classical concept that disturbed function is the result and not a cause of a changed morphological substratum.

An illustrative example is the case of von Bergmann (30), who as early as 1913 claimed that peptic ulcers probably result from a chronic gastric neurosis caused by emotional factors, yet fourteen years later felt it necessary to revise his views and to return to a more conservative attitude recommending great reservation regarding the diagnosis of an "organ neurosis." He expressed his belief that in most such cases further research would disclose organic causes (31).

For a long time the scientific credo in medicine has been that further histological studies would reveal an anatomical basis for all so-called functional disturbances. Today we feel that in many cases a thorough investigation of the patient's life history might reveal the origins of early functional disturbances before the disturbance of function has produced histologically discernible organic changes. The resistance to this concept is based on the erroneous dogma that disturbed function is *always* the result of disturbed structure and on a disregard of the reverse causal sequence.

At present it is difficult to say which organic diseases follow this latter etiological pattern. It is most probable that in the great chapter of medicine which might be called "Chronic Diseases of Unknown Origin," many will fall into this category. In many endocrine disorders chronic emotional disturbances are probably important etiological factors. This is clearly indicated in cases of toxic goiter, the onset of which can frequently be traced to emotional traumata. The influence of emotions on carbohydrate metabolism makes it possible that in the development of diabetes, emotional factors may play an important causative role.

This functional theory of organic disorders is essentially the recognition, apart from acute *external* causative factors, of chronic *internal* causes of disease. In other words, many chronic disturbances are not caused primarily by external, mechanical, or chemical factors or by microorganisms, but by the continuous functional stress arising during the everyday life of the individual in his struggle for existence. Those emotional conflicts which psychoanalysis recognizes as the basis of psychoneuroses and as the ultimate cause of certain functional and organic disorders, arise during our daily life in our contact with the environment. Fear, aggression, guilt, frustrated wishes, if repressed, result in permanent chronic emotional tensions which disturb the functions of the vegetative organs. Because of the complications of our social life, many emotions cannot be expressed and relieved freely through voluntary activities but remain repressed and are eventually diverted into inappropriate channels. Instead of being expressed in voluntary innervations, they influence the vegetative functions, such as digestion, respiration, and circulation. Just as countries thwarted in their external political ambitions often experience internal social upheavals, so the human organism too may show a disturbance of its internal politics, of its vegetative functions, if its relation to the world is disturbed.

There is much evidence that just as certain pathological microorganisms have a specific affinity for certain organs, so also certain emotional conflicts possess specificities and accordingly tend to afflict certain internal organs. Inhibited rage seems to have a specific relationship to the cardiovascular system (Cannon; Fahrenkamp; Hill; K. Menninger; K. Menninger and W. Menninger; Wolfe; Dunbar; Draper; Saul; Alexander; Dunbar—43, 81, 118, 152, 154, 256, 71, 67, 202, 7, 73); dependent help-seeking tendencies seem to have a specific relationship to the functions of nutrition (Ruesch, et al.; Kapp, et al.; Alexander; Bacon; Levey—199, 129, 9, 20, 136). Again, a conflict between sexual wishes and dependent tendencies seems to have a specific influence upon the respiratory functions [1] (French, Alexander, et al.—89). The increasing knowledge of the relations of emotions to normal and disturbed body functions requires the modern physician to regard emotional conflicts as just as real and concrete as visible microorganisms. The main contribution of psychoanalysis to medicine has been to add to the optical microscope a psycho-

[1] The question of specificity of psychological factors will be discussed further on pages 68 ff.

logical microscope—that is to say, a psychological technique by which the emotional life of the patient can be subjected to detailed investigation.

This psychosomatic approach to the problems of life and disease brings internal physiological processes into synthesis with the individual's relations to his social environment. It gives a scientific basis to empirical observations such as, for example, that a patient often shows marvelous recovery if he is removed from his family environment or if he interrupts his everyday occupations and thus is relieved of those emotional conflicts which stem from familial or professional relations. Detailed knowledge of the relationship between emotional life and body processes extends the function of the physician: the physical and mental care of the patient can be co-ordinated into an integral whole of medical therapy. This is the real meaning of "psychosomatic medicine."

Chapter VII

Methodological Considerations Concerning the Psychosomatic Approach

THE TERM "psychosomatic" has been subjected to much criticism, chiefly because it seems to imply a dichotomy between mind and body. This dichotomy is precisely what the psychosomatic point of view tries to avoid. And if we understand psychic phenomena as the subjective aspect of certain physiological (brain) processes, this dichotomy disappears. Besides, most terms referring to a complex subject matter are ambiguous. To mention only one, the term "psychoanalysis," now so firmly established, has from the linguistic point of view a superfluous "o" in it, and—what is more important—it does not indicate that the aim of psychoanalytic therapy is synthetic rather than analytic, namely to increase the integrative capacities of the ego. In a field as complex as the one under discussion any expression we might choose, such as "dynamic medicine" or "the holistic approach" needs definition. The concepts which are associated today with the term "psychosomatic" have penetrated medical thought and literature. The expression should be retained but should be defined clearly and unequivocally. Once we agree precisely upon what we mean it makes little difference what symbol we use.

The term "psychosomatic" should be used only to indicate a *method of approach* both in research and in therapy, namely the simultaneous and co-ordinated use of somatic—i.e., physiological, anatomical, pharmacological, surgical, and dietary—methods and concepts on the one hand, and psychological methods and concepts on the other. Emphasis is placed upon the qualification "co-ordinated use," indicating that the two methods are applied in the conceptual framework of causal sequences. To make this more concrete, the study of gastric secretion may be restricted to physiological methods by which the local process is studied. It may also include the physiological study of nervous impulses controlling gastric secretion. This is still purely somatic research. The psychosomatic study of gastric secretion, however, approaches not only one part of this complex process but its totality and therefore includes central cortical stimuli which influence gastric secretion and which cannot be described or investigated except by psychological methods. For example, nostalgic longings and the desire to receive help and affection also stimulate gastric activity. They represent certain brain processes, yet they can be described meaningfully only in psychological terms because receptive longings cannot at this time be identified by biochemical, electrical, or any other non-psychological technique. These brain processes are subjectively perceived as emotions and can be conveyed to others by speech. They can therefore be studied psychologically, and, what is more important, they can be studied adequately *only* by psychological means.

The question may be raised, then, as to whether the psychosomatic approach should be considered as a transitory method which will be abandoned as soon as we are able by improved electroencephalography and other physiological techniques to study those brain processes which today yield only to psychological methods. While this question cannot be answered with certainty, it appears probable that brain processes pertaining to interpersonal relationships can be adequately described only in psychological and sociological terms. Even improved physiological methods will allow the study of processes within the organism itself only. A biochemical formula describing a receptive longing somewhere in the cortex will never account for the interpersonal circumstances under which this longing arose or became intensified, nor will it indicate those changes in interpersonal relations by which its intensity can be reduced and thus its harmful effect upon stomach activity alleviated.

Another controversial question is the diagnostic or classificatory concept of "psychosomatic disease," proposed by Halliday (110, 111, 112, 115). Such diseases would include peptic ulcer, rheumatoid arthritis, hyperthyroidism, essential hypertension, and many others. This view is based on the assumption that in these diseases the outstanding etiological factor is psychological. All available evidence, however, points to multicausal explanations in all branches of medicine (Alexander—12). We are no longer satisfied to say that tuberculosis is caused by exposure to the bacillus of Koch but recognize that specific and non-specific immunity, the resistance of the organism to infection, is a complex phenomenon which may depend partly on emotional factors. Accordingly, tuberculosis is a psychosomatic disease. And conversely, the merely psychogenic explanation of such diseases as peptic ulcer cannot be defended in view of the fact that the typical emotional constellations found in patients suffering from ulcer are also observed in a large number of patients who do not suffer from ulcers. Local or general somatic factors, as yet ill defined, must be assumed, and only the coexistence of both kinds of factors, emotional and somatic, can account for ulcer formation. Equally important is the fact that in different cases the relative importance of somatic and emotional factors varies to a high degree. Multicausality and the varying distribution of psychological and non-psychological factors from case to case invalidates the concept of "psychosomatic disease" as a specific diagnostic group. Theoretically every disease is psychosomatic, since emotional factors influence all body processes through nervous and humoral pathways.

The following factors may be of etiological importance in disease:

$$D \text{ (disease)} = f \text{ (function of)} \left\{ a . b . c . d . e . g . h . i . j .... n \right.$$

a — hereditary constitution
b — birth injuries
c — organic diseases of infancy which increase the vulnerability of certain organs
d — nature of infant care (weaning habits, toilet training, sleeping arrangements, etc.)
e — accidental physical traumatic experiences of infancy and childhood
g — accidental emotional traumatic experiences of infancy and childhood
h — emotional climate of family and specific personality traits of parents and siblings
i — later physical injuries
j — later emotional experiences in intimate personal and occupational relations

These factors in different proportions are of etiological significance in all diseases. The psychosomatic point of view added the factors d, g, h, and j to the other factors, which have long been given attention in medicine. Only the consideration of all these categories and their interaction can give a complete etiological picture.

In this connection it should be emphasized as a further methodological postulate that psychosomatic investigation requires a detailed and precise description of psychological sequences just as it requires a precise observation of the correlated physiological processes. Detailed physiological studies which are correlated with haphazard impressionistic psychological descriptions cannot contribute to our better knowledge of etiology. To describe disturbed heart activity precisely and to explain it as being caused by nervousness without adequate description of emotional and ideational content is meaningless.

Chapter VIII

Fundamental Principles of the Psychosomatic Approach

1. PSYCHOGENESIS

THE PROBLEM of psychogenesis is linked up with the ancient dichotomy of psyche versus soma. Psychological and somatic phenomena take place in the same organism and are merely two aspects of the same process. In the living organism certain physiological processes are perceived subjectively as feelings, ideas, and strivings. As has been pointed out before, these physiological processes can best be approached by psychological methods which deal with the communication of the subjectively perceived physiological processes through speech. Fundamentally, therefore, the object of psychological studies is no different from that of physiology; the two differ only in the manner of approach.

It is important that we state specifically what is meant by "psychogenesis." First, let us take an example. In the case of emotionally caused elevation of blood pressure, psychogenesis does not mean that the contraction of the blood vessels is effected by some non-somatic mechanism. Rage consists in physiological processes which take place somewhere in the central nervous system. The physiological effect of rage consists of a chain of events in which every link can be described, at least theoretically, in physiological terms. The distinctive feature of psychogenic factors such as emotions or ideas and fantasies is that they *can also* be studied psychologically through introspection or by verbal communication from those in whom these physiological processes take place. Verbal communication is therefore one of the most potent instruments of psychology and, by the same token, of psychosomatic research. When we speak of psychogenesis we refer to physiological processes consisting of central excitations in the nervous system which can be studied by psychological methods because they are perceived subjectively in the form of emotions, ideas, or wishes. Psychosomatic research deals with processes in which certain links in the causal chain lend themselves, at the present state of our knowledge, more readily to a study by psychological than by physiological methods, since the detailed investigation of emotions as brain processes is not far enough advanced. Even when the physiological basis of psychological phenomena is better known, it is not likely that we can dispense with their psychological study. It is hardly conceivable that the different moves of two chess players would ever be more clearly understood in biochemical or neurophysiological than in psychological terms.

2. PHYSIOLOGICAL FUNCTIONS AFFECTED BY PSYCHOLOGICAL INFLUENCES

These can be divided into three main categories:
(a) Voluntary behavior.
(b) Expressive innervations.
(c) Vegetative responses to emotional states.

CO-ORDINATED VOLUNTARY BEHAVIOR

Voluntary behavior is carried out under the influence of psychological motivations. For example, upon the perception of hunger certain co-ordinated movements are carried out which are suited to obtaining food and relieving hunger. Each step is undertaken under the influence of certain psychological processes. One remembers, for example, where the food has been stored, or the place where the restaurant is, and so forth. These intermediary psychological links may be simple, such as remembering that there is food in the refrigerator. Or they may be quite complicated: A hobo awakens in the morning with a feeling of hunger and has no money in his pocket. He must first offer his services to someone, who accepts them, and only after payment for his work can he relieve his hunger. In our complex civilization a great part of our lives consists in preparation to become economically productive members of society in order to secure the basic biological needs of food, shelter, etc. The life history of everyone can be considered, therefore, a complex psychosomatic process, goal-directed voluntary behavior, executed under the direction of certain psychological influences (motivations).

The dynamic system of psychological forces whose function is to carry out this complicated task of co-ordination is called the *ego*. Failures of its functions give rise to the different forms of psychoneuroses and psychoses. These disturbances belong to the field of psychiatry proper.

EXPRESSIVE INNERVATIONS

These are physiological processes, such as weeping, sighing, laughing, blushing, gesticulating, and grimacing, which take place under the influence of specific emotional tensions. All these complex movements express certain emotions and at the same time relieve a specific emotional tension, sadness, self-pity, humor, and so forth. These expressive innervations do not pursue any utilitarian goals; they do not serve the satisfaction of any basic biological need; their only function is the relief of an emotional tension. Laughter, for example, occurs under the influence of certain emotional situations which have a comical effect. Some of the best minds—Bergson, Lipps, and Freud, to mention only a few—have attempted to define what constitutes a comical effect by finding a common denominator for those interpersonal situations to which laughter is the universal response. A tall and a short fellow are walking side by side when suddenly the tall one stumbles and falls. The effect is highly comical. The more haughtily the tall one was walking, the greater is the comical effect of his sudden fall. Here it is easy to recognize that the onlooker gives vent in his laughter to some pent-up malice; he laughs at the expense of the tall fellow. Everyone has in childhood sometimes envied and resented the adults with whom he tried so hard to keep up while trotting beside them on the street. They were giants who could push us around at their desire, and we were completely helpless before them. Every onlooker identifies himself unconsciously with the small fellow who unperturbedly walks on while his tall companion suddenly lies prostrated on the ground. In a masterly fashion Freud showed that hidden hostile tendencies constitute one aspect of the comical effect (95).

Still other subtle psychological factors must be present in order to precipitate laughter, this highly complex phenomenon consisting of the spasmodic contractions of the diaphragm and of the facial muscles. It is not my purpose to elaborate the finer psychological details. I select laughter as an example to demonstrate two important facts: first, the complex and specific nature of the psychological stimuli which motivate such expressive movements as laughter; and, second, the discharge nature of this kind of innervation which does not serve any utilitarian goal. In a classroom a fly lights on the bald head of the teacher. For a while the boys control their urge to laugh. Then one of them begins to snicker, and the next moment the whole class erupts in uncontrollable laughter. Obviously the aggressive impulses against the teacher pent up in every schoolboy find a sudden eruptive release. The laughter takes its course; a certain amount of muscular energy is required to relieve the psychological tension. Similarly, weeping, sighing, and frowning have no utility; they serve merely to discharge specific emotional tensions.

From the point of view of physiology, the sexual phenomena belong in this category. They are also discharge phenomena serving the relief of specific instinctual tensions.

Pathological alterations involving such expressive processes belong customarily to the field of psychiatry. Emotions which are repressed because they are in conflict with the standards of the personality cannot be discharged through the ordinary channels of expressive innervations. The patient has to invent his own individual expressive innervations in the form of conversion symptoms which serve partially to discharge the repressed emotions and partially as defenses against their direct expression. Sometimes the discharge takes place through the usual appropriate expressive processes such as occurs in the case of hysterical weeping and laughter. Here, the underlying emotions are repressed and the patient does not know why he weeps or laughs. Because of the dissociation of the expressive movements from the underlying emotion, they cannot relieve the tension. Hence the uncontrollable and prolonged nature of hysterical laughter or weeping.

VEGETATIVE RESPONSES TO EMOTIONAL STATES

This group of responses consists in visceral reactions to emotional stimuli and is of particular significance for internal medicine and other medical specialties. The psychosomatic approach in medicine originated in the study of vegetative disturbances which develop under certain emotional states. Before undertaking a discussion of the vegetative disturbances, however, we have to describe the normal bodily responses to emotions; these serve as the physiological bases of the various disturbances affecting the different vegetative organs.

The total functioning of the nervous system can be understood as being aimed at maintaining conditions within the organism in a constant state (homeostasis). The nervous system achieves this task by the principle of the division of labor. Whereas the voluntary central nervous system is entrusted with the regulation of the relations to the external world, the autonomic nervous system controls the internal affairs of the organism, i.e. the internal vegetative processes. The parasympathetic division of the autonomic nervous system is more explicitly concerned with conservation and upbuilding, i.e. with anabolic processes. Its anabolic influence manifests itself in functions such as the stimulation of gastrointestinal digestive activity and the storing of sugar in the liver. Its conserving and protecting function expresses itself, for example, in contractions of the pupil as protection against light, or in the spasm of the bronchioli as protection against irritating substances.

As was postulated by Cannon (43), the main function of the sympathetic portions of the autonomic nervous system is the regulation of internal vegetative functions in relation to external activities, particularly in emergency situations. In other words, the sympathetic nervous system is involved in the preparation of the organism for fight and flight by modifying the vegetative processes in a way most useful in emergency situations. In preparation for fight and flight, as well as during such activities, it inhibits all anabolic processes; thus it becomes an inhibitor of gastrointestinal activity. It stimulates heart and lung action, however, and changes the distribution of the blood, driving it from the splanchnic area to the muscles and lungs and the cerebrum, where an augmented supply of energy is needed for their increased action. At the same time the blood pressure rises, carbohydrates are mobilized from their depots, and the adrenal medulla is stimulated. To a high degree the sympathetic and parasympathetic actions are antagonistic.

The generalization may be made that under parasympathetic preponderance the individual withdraws from his external problems into a merely vegetative existence, whereas under sympathetic stimulation he neglects or inhibits his peaceful functions of upbuilding and growth and turns all his attention toward facing his problems in relation to the external environment.

The internal economy of the organism during effort and relaxation behaves as a nation does in war and in peace. War economy means priorities for war goods and prohibition of certain peacetime productions. Tanks are produced instead of passenger cars, munitions are produced instead of luxury goods. In the organism, the emotional state of preparedness corresponds to war economy and relaxation to peace economy, as certain organ systems which are needed in the emergency become stimulated while the others are inhibited.

In neurotic disturbances of the vegetative functions, this harmony between external situation and internal vegetative processes is disturbed. The disturbance may take different forms.

Only a limited number of conditions have been thoroughly studied from the psychodynamic point of view. In general, the emotional disturbances of vegetative functions can be divided into two main categories. These two categories correspond to the two basic emotional attitudes described above:

(1) Preparation for fight, or flight, in emergency.

(2) Withdrawal from outwardly directed activity.

(1) The disturbances belonging to the first group are the results of inhibition or repression of self-assertive, hostile impulses. Because the impulses are repressed or inhibited, the corresponding behavior (fight or flight) is never consummated. And yet the organism is physiologically in a constant state of preparedness. In other words, although the vegetative processes have been mobilized for concentrated aggressive activity,

they are not brought to full-fledged action. The result is that the chronic state of preparedness persists in the organism together with those physiological reactions which are normally needed in an emergency situation, such as increased heart rate, heightened blood pressure, or dilatation of the blood vessels in the skeletal muscles, an increased mobilization of carbohydrates, and increased metabolism.

In a normal individual, these physiological changes are only temporary, lasting only so long as the need for increased effort persists. After fight or flight, or whenever the task requiring effort is accomplished, the organism reposes and the physiological processes return to normal. This is not the case, however, when, following the activation of the vegetative processes involved in the preparation for action, no action takes place. If this occurs repeatedly, some of the above-described adaptive physiological responses remain chronic. Various forms of cardiac symptoms exemplify these phenomena. These symptoms are reactions to neurotic anxiety and repressed or inhibited rage. In essential hypertension the increased blood pressure is chronically sustained under the influence of pent-up and never fully relieved emotions, just as would happen temporarily under the influence of freely expressed rage in normal persons. Emotional influences upon the regulatory mechanisms of carbohydrate metabolism probably play a significant role in diabetes mellitus. Chronically increased muscle tension brought about by sustained aggressive impulses appear to be a pathogenic factor in rheumatoid arthritis. The influence of this type of emotion upon endocrine functions can be observed in thyrotoxicosis. Vascular responses to emotional tensions play an important role in certain forms of headaches. In all these examples, certain phases of the vegetative preparation for concentrated action are chronically sustained because the underlying motivating forces are neurotically inhibited and are not released in appropriate action.

(2) A second group of neurotic persons react to the necessity for concentrated self-assertive behavior with an emotional withdrawal from action into a dependent state. Instead of facing the emergency, their first impulse is to turn for help as they did when they were helpless children. This retreat from action to an attitude which is characteristic for the organism during relaxation may be termed "vegetative retreat." A common example of this phenomenon is a man who develops diarrhea when in danger instead of acting in an appropriate manner. He "has no guts." Instead of acting to meet the emergency he performs a vegetative accomplishment for which he received praise from his mother when he was an infant. This type of neurotic vegetative response constitutes a more complete withdrawal from action than those discussed in the first group. That group make the required adaptive vegetative responses; their disturbance consists only in the fact that their vegetative preparation for action under sympathetic or humoral stimulation becomes chronic. The second group of patients reacts paradoxically: instead of preparing for outwardly directed action, they retreat into a vegetative condition which is just the reverse of what is appropriate.

This psychophysiological process can be demonstrated by observations such as I made upon a patient suffering from a gastric neurosis connected with chronic hyperacidity. This patient, whenever he saw a moving picture in which a hero was fighting enemies or was engaged in activities of an aggressive, dangerous character, reacted with acute heartburn. In his fantasy, he identified himself with the hero. This aroused anxiety, however, and he retreated from fight to seek security and help. As we will see later, such dependent desires for security and help are intimately connected with the wish to be fed, and so produce increased activity of the stomach. This patient behaved paradoxically in so far as his vegetative responses go, because just when he had to fight, his stomach began to overfunction and prepare itself for the intake of food. Even in animal life, the enemy must first be defeated before it can be devoured.

The large group of so-called *functional disturbances of the gastrointestinal tract* belong here. All forms of nervous indigestion, nervous diarrhea, cardiospasm, various forms of colitis, and certain forms of constipation are illustrative. These gastrointestinal responses to emotional stress can be considered as being based on "regressive patterns," because they represent a revival of bodily responses to emotional tensions which are characteristic for the infant. One of the first emotional tensions perceived by the child is hunger, which is relieved by oral incorporation followed by the feeling of satiation. Oral incorporation thus becomes an early pattern for relieving the unpleasant tension caused by an unsatisfied need. This old way of resolving a painful tension may be revived in adults in a neurotic condition or under acute emotional stress. A married woman reported that whenever she felt thwarted or rejected by her husband she found herself sucking her thumbs. This phenomenon truly deserves the expression "regression." The nervous habit of smoking or chewing in a state of suspended or impatient expectation is based on the same type of regressive pattern. Emotionally precipitated responses in bowel function are similar regressive phenomena and may occur under extreme emotional stress even in otherwise healthy individuals.

Furthermore, this type of emotional mechanism has an important etiological significance in conditions in which gross morphological changes develop such as peptic ulcer and ulcerative colitis. In addition to gastrointestinal disturbances, certain forms of fatigue states which are associated with disturbance of the carbohydrate metabolism belong in this group of neurotic responses. Likewise, the psychological component in bronchial asthma represents a retreat from action into a dependent, help-seeking attitude. All the disturbed functions in this group are stimulated by the parasympathetic nervous system, and are inhibited by sympathetic stimulation. One is inclined to assume in the first category of vegetative responses a sympathetic preponderance and in the latter group a parasympathetic preponderance in autonomic balance. This assumption, however, does not take into consideration the fact that every displacement of autonomic equilibrium produces instantaneous compensatory reactions. The disturbance at its onset may well be caused by an excess of sympathetic or parasympathetic stimulation. Soon, however, the picture becomes complicated by counter-regulatory mechanisms aimed at restoring the homeostatic equilibrium. In all vegetative functions both divisions of the autonomic nervous system are involved, and once a disturbance has been initiated it is no longer possible to ascribe the ensuing symptoms exclusively to either sympathetic or parasympathetic influences. Only at the onset can the disturbing stimulus be identified with one or the other division of the autonomic nervous system. It must also be borne in mind that the homeostatic regulations often overshoot their mark and the overcompensatory response may overshadow the originally disturbing stimulus. The two portions of the autonomic nervous system are antagonistic in their function, yet in every vegetative process they collaborate, just as the extensor and flexor muscles, though they have antagonistic functions, co-operate in every motion of the extremities.

SUMMARY

Confronting the herein-discussed physiological facts with the psychoanalytic theory of neuroses in general and the previously advanced views of vegetative neurosis in particular, we come to the following consistent picture. Every neurosis consists, to a certain degree, of withdrawal from action, in the substitution of autoplastic processes for action (Freud). In psychoneuroses without physical symptoms, motor activity is replaced by psychological activity, by acting in fantasy instead of reality. The division of labor in the central nervous system, however, is not disturbed. The psychoneurotic symptoms are based on the activity of the central nervous system, the function of which is the control of external relationships. This holds true also for conversion hysteria. Here, too, the symptoms are localized in the voluntary and sensoryperceptive system, which deals with the external affairs of the organism. Every neurotic disturbance of vegetative function, however, consists in a disturbance of the division of labor within the nervous system. In these cases outward-directed action is omitted and the unrelieved emotional tension induces chronic internal vegetative changes. In those cases which are based on sympathetic preponderance this disturbance of the division of labor is not so thoroughgoing as in those in which a parasympathetic excitation prevails. Sympathetic functions, as we have seen, take an intermediary position between internal vegetative functions and outwardly directed action; they tune up and change the vegetative functions in a way that is conducive to action directed toward the solution of external problems. In disturbances where there is a sympathetic hyperactivity, the organism does not go into action, although it undergoes all those preparatory changes which are conducive to action and necessary for it. If this were followed by action, the process would be normal. The neurotic nature of the condition is that the whole physiological process never comes to consummation.

We see a more complete withdrawal from the solution of external problems in those disorders which develop under parasympathetic preponderance. Here the unconscious psychological material which is connected with the symptom corresponds to a withdrawal to an early vegetative dependence upon the mother organism. The patient suffering from gastrointestinal symptoms reacts to the need for action with paradoxical vegetative responses: for example, he prepares himself to be fed instead of to fight.

The division of vegetative symptoms into these two groups is only a preliminary step toward a solution of the question of emotional specificity in organ neuroses. The next problem is to understand those specific factors which could account for the choice of the organ function within the larger division of parasympathetic or sympathetic action, to explain why unconscious aggressive fighting tendencies, if repressed, lead in some cases to chronic hypertension and in other cases to palpitation or to a disturbance of the carbohydrate metabolism or to chronic constipation, and why passive regressive tendencies lead to gastric symptoms in some instances and to diarrhea and asthma in others.

Psychodynamically the two types of neurotic responses in vegetative functions can be represented by the diagram shown in Figure I.

Whenever the expression of competitive, aggressive, and hostile attitudes is inhibited in voluntary behavior, the sympathetic adrenal system is in sustained excitation. The vegetative symptoms result from the sustained sympathetic excitation, which persists because no consummation of the fight or flight reaction takes place in the field of co-ordinated voluntary behavior, as exemplified by the patient suffering from essential hypertension who in his overt behavior appears inhibited and under excessive control. Likewise in migraine headache, the painful attack may terminate within a few minutes after the patient becomes conscious of his rage and gives open expression to it.[1]

In those cases in which the gratification of help-seeking, regressive tendencies is absent from overt behavior either because of internal denial of these tendencies or because of external circumstances, the vegetative responses are apt to manifest themselves in dysfunctions which are the results of an increased parasympathetic activity. Examples are the overtly hyperactive, energetic peptic ulcer patient who does

[1] See page 160.

Figure I.

Schematic illustration of the concept of specificity in the etiology of the disturbances of vegetative functions

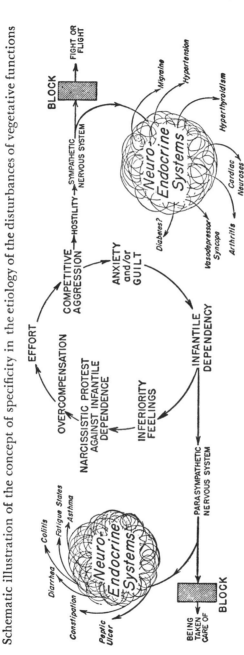

This diagram shows the two kinds of vegetative responses to emotional states. On the right side of the diagram are shown those conditions which may develop when the expression of the hostile aggressive impulse (fight or flight) is blocked and is absent in overt behavior; on the left side appear those conditions which develop when the dependent help-seeking tendencies are blocked.

not allow gratification of his dependent needs, and the patient who develops chronic incapacitating fatigue whenever he tries to engage in some activity requiring concentrated effort. In other words, these vegetative symptoms are initiated by a sustained excitation of the parasympathetic branch of the autonomic nervous system induced by sustained emotional tension which cannot find relief in overt co-ordinated voluntary behavior.

These correlations between symptoms and unconscious attitudes cannot be extended simply to a correlation between overt personality features and symptoms. Moreover, a combination of both types of reaction may be observed in the same person in different periods of life and in some cases even simultaneously.[1]

3. THE PROBLEM OF THE SPECIFICITY OF EMOTIONAL FACTORS IN SOMATIC DISTURBANCES

The views proposed in the preceding pages are based on what is called the theory of specificity. According to this theory, physiological responses to emotional stimuli, both normal and morbid, vary according to the nature of the precipitating emotional state. Laughter is the response to merriment, weeping to sorrow; sighing expresses relief or despair, and blushing expresses embarrassment. The vegetative responses to different emotional stimuli vary also according to the quality of the emotions. Every emotional state has its own physiological syndrome. Increased blood pressure and accelerated heart action are a constituent part of rage and fear. Increased stomach secretion may be a regressive response to an emergency. Attacks of asthma are correlated with an unconscious suppressed impulse to cry for the mother's help.

[1] The distinction made here between sympathetic and parasympathetic preponderance is not related at all to Eppinger's and Hess's concepts of sympaticotonic and vago-tonic constitutions, since sympathetic or parasympathetic preponderance is not a constant characteristic of a person, but only of transient conditions.

How specific the physiological responses to various emotional stimuli are is still an open question. The proposed theory differentiates principally between two attitudes: (1) preparation to deal with the anxiety-producing situation by meeting it actively and (2) retreat from it to increased dependence like the small child who turns to the mother for help instead of trying to meet the emergency himself. In accord with Cannon's (43) concepts, the first type of emotional attitude goes with increased sympathetic, the second with increased parasympathetic excitation. Within these two large categories specific responses to different emotions can be distinguished. These will be discussed in the following chapters.

The older view still has its adherents—namely, that there is no specific correlation between the nature of emotional stress and its physical sequelae. This concept maintains that any emotion may contribute to any organic disturbance and the local vulnerability of the affected organ is responsible for the localization of a disease. The theory of emotional specificity does not, however, disregard other non-emotional factors which may determine the type of physiological response.[1] The constitution and the history of the organ system involved are also important influences which contribute to its specific susceptibility to emotional stimuli.

The controversy concerning the specificity of the psychodynamic factors operative in vegetative disturbances is obscured by the fact that the significant psychological influences, such as anxiety, repressed hostile and erotic impulses, frustration or dependent cravings, inferiority and guilt feelings, are present in all these disorders. It is not the presence of any one or more of these psychological factors that is specific but the presence of the dynamic configuration in which they appear. This type of specificity is similar to that found in stereochemistry. The constituent parts in the different organic compounds are the same atoms: carbon, hydrogen, oxygen,

[1] See discussion of etiological factors on page 52.

and nitrogen; they are combined, however, in a great variety of structural patterns, and each combination represents a substance of highly specific quality. Further, there is specificity in the manner in which a psychological motivating force may express itself. Hostility can be expressed in physical attack, be it via the extremities or by soiling, spitting, etc., or by verbal invectives, destructive fantasies, or other less direct modes of attack. The physiological responses will vary accordingly. The wish to be taken care of as seen in vegetative retreats may appear as the wish to be fed, caressed, carried around, catered to, praised, encouraged, or helped by others in any of a variety of other ways. As will be shown in detail in reference to the different vegetative disorders, the psychological content together with the dynamic configuration of these motivating forces determines the physiological functions that will be activated or inhibited. A valuable approach to the study of the specific physiological responses to psychological stimuli has been used by French. Since "every integrated activity involves the functional excitation, now of one organ, now of another, according to the particular pattern of activity," the repressed motivations in dreams may express themselves by bodily functions which correspond to the psychological stimuli (88).

The precise reconstruction of the specific psychodynamic configurations characteristic of the various vegetative disturbances is most difficult and requires a painstaking comparative anamnestic study of a great number of patients suffering from the same type of disorder. The data obtained by such studies must then be compared with detailed psychoanalytic observations made on a smaller number of cases. Some of the specific psychodynamic patterns characteristic for various diseases are presented at the ends of the chapters in the second part of this book.[1]

---

[1] See pages 115, 128, 153, 184, and 208–209.

4. PERSONALITY TYPE AND DISEASE

The concept that certain personality types are predisposed to certain diseases has been ever present in medical thought. When medicine was based on clinical observation alone the frequent occurrence of certain diseases in persons of definite physical or mental habitus was often noted by observant physicians. The significance of this fact, however, was completely unknown. The good clinician prided himself on knowing these correlations from lifelong experience. He knew that the lean, longitudinal, narrow-chested person was more inclined to tuberculosis than the rotund, robust type and that the latter was more apt to suffer a cerebral hemorrhage. Such correlations between disease and physical build were paralleled by correlations between personality traits and certain diseases. Expressions like "melancholia" reveal the intuitive knowledge of the frequency of depressive traits among sufferers from gall-bladder disturbance. (melas = black, chole = gall). Balzac (21) in his *Cousin Pons,* one of the first psychosomatic novels ever written, gives a masterful description of a bachelor, who developed first melancholia and later a gall-bladder disease. The inclination of diabetics toward culinary pleasures and the relationship of disturbances of the heart to anxiety have been commonly known. In this country, clinicians like Alvarez, George Draper, Eli Moschcowitz (18, 69, 168, 169, 170), and others have contributed valuable observations of this kind which will be discussed in greater detail in subsequent chapters. The concept of the peptic-ulcer personality, the hard-driving go-getter type, has been advanced by Alvarez (19). Draper (68) recognized that, underneath, many of the peptic-ulcer patients showed dependent and, as he expressed it, feminine characteristics.

Another fertile field for the correlation of personality traits with disease pictures is in endocrine diseases, such as hyper-

and hypothyroidism. The high-strung, excitable, sensitive patient suffering from toxic goiter is in sharp contrast to the slow, phlegmatic, dull person with hypothyroidism.

Most of these observations were of more or less anecdotal nature until Dunbar (75) applied the modern methods of psychodynamic diagnosis to this fertile field. In her "profile studies" she describes certain statistical correlations between disease and personality type. The external personality patterns which can be described by her method vary to such a degree among patients suffering from the same disease that at best one could speak only of certain more or less significant statistical frequencies. The fact that exceptions are so numerous in itself indicates that most of these correlations are not truly causal in nature.

Perhaps the most valid of her profiles is that of the coronary patient. According to Dunbar such a patient is usually a consistently striving person of great control and persistence, aiming at success and accomplishment. He is a long-term planner: he is often distinguished-looking. He displays a high degree of what Freud called the "reality principle," the capacity for postponing and subordinating actions to long-term goals. Dunbar impressively contrasted such patients with fracture patients who are prone to accidents. These are impulsive, unsystematic, adventurous persons living for the present and not for the future. They are inclined to act on the spur of the moment and frequently manifest ill-controlled hostility against persons in authority; at the same time their behavior is motivated by guilt feelings and shows a tendency toward self-punishment and failure. These accident-prone persons are found commonly among the hobo types, the happy-go-lucky people who cannot tolerate discipline, either external authority or the internal regulative influence of reason.[1]

The correlation between a tendency toward impulsive action and a lack of tolerance for external or internal disci-

[1] See pages 209 ff.

pline on the one hand and accident-proneness on the other appears to constitute a definite causal relationship. It is easily understandable that an impulsive person, full of hostility and guilt feelings, will be inclined to have accidents. His actions are rash and he has at the same time also a tendency toward self-punishment and suffering. He is incautious and at the same time is inclined to pay a price in the form of physical injury for his aggressions.

The relationship between certain personality types and coronary disease appears to be much more complex. The frequency of coronary accidents among patients in such professional groups as physicians, priests, lawyers, executives, and persons who carry great responsibilities is well known among clinicians. In this sense coronary disease appears almost as an occupational disease. It might well be that a certain type of living, certain types of mental exertion, create somatic conditions conducive to certain progressive changes in the vascular system resulting ultimately in coronary disease. The true correlation may be not between personality make-up and coronary disease but between the mode of living and the disease. Dunbar's finding would then be explained from the fact that certain personality types are more inclined to assume such responsible occupations. It is a secondary correlation and not a directly causal one. A pseudo correlation of this type is Dunbar's statement that coronary patients are frequently distinguished-looking. The distinguished look is obviously due to the fact that these persons are often educated, professional people. The external appearance probably has little to do with coronary disease itself.

This type of pseudo correlation can be illustrated with the following example. One could predict with certainty that in Italy among industrial workers there are more blonds than among agricultural workers. This correlation only reveals the fact that the industrial area of Italy is in the North, where more blond people live, than in southern Italy, where people are swarthy and where they are engaged mostly in agricultural work. This correlation does not reveal any mystical relationship or affinity between industrial work and blondness. As long as the more detailed mechanisms between emotional factors and organic diseases are not known, the establishment of certain external correlations between superficially observable personality features and diseases is of limited significance.

Another kind of correlation between personality factors and disease has greater significance. Thorough psychodynamic investigations have shown that certain disturbances of vegetative functions can be directly correlated with specific emotional states rather than with superficial personality configurations as described in personality profiles. For example, chronically sustained hostile impulses can be correlated with a chronic elevation of the blood pressure while dependent help-seeking trends go with increased gastric secretion. These emotional states, however, may occur in a great number of very different personalities. It is true that the go-getter type who represses and overcompensates for dependent tendencies is commonly found among peptic-ulcer patients. Some of them, however, do not show this personality structure at all; they do not repress their help-demanding attitudes but are constantly frustrated in their gratification by external circumstances.[1] These patients are not hard-driving, responsibility-loving persons; they are openly dependent or demanding. We know by now that it is of secondary importance whether or not the dependent tendency is thwarted by internal factors such as pride or by external factors such as a cold, rejecting wife. The significant correlation is between the wish to receive love and help and the activity of the stomach, no matter whether this wish is thwarted through external circumstances or by pride which prevents a person from accepting external help. Likewise the nuclear conflict in asthma cases is well

[1] See further discussion on page 103.

circumscribed and distinct: fear of separation from the mother or her substitute. However, the overt personalities may vary markedly. The characteristic emotional pattern of the asthmatic may occur in a great variety of contrasting personality types who defend themselves against the fear of separation by various emotional devices.

A mysterious and vague correlation between personality and disease does not exist; there is a distinct correlation between certain emotional constellations and certain vegetative innervations. Whatever correlation is found between personality type and somatic disease is only of relative statistical validity and often incidental. Under given cultural conditions certain defenses against emotional conflicts appear more frequently than others. Our culture, for example, puts great emphasis on independence and personal accomplishment; hence the frequency among peptic-ulcer patients of the hyperactive go-getter type. This surface picture is but a defense (overcompensation) against deep-seated dependent longings and has no direct correlation with the ulcer formation. The true psychosomatic correlations are between emotional constellations and vegetative responses.

5. RELATION OF NERVOUS AND HORMONAL MECHANISMS

As mentioned above, the participation of the two branches of the autonomic nervous system in various symptoms cannot be isolated precisely, since, although they are antagonists in their action, they collaborate in the regulation of every vegetative function. Moreover, owing to homeostatic equilibration, an initial shift in either sympathetic or parasympathetic stimulation may be overcompensated in the opposite direction. The longer a disturbance prevails, the more complex becomes the autonomic participation. The picture is further complicated by the fact that in chronic conditions the neurogenic mechanisms become less important and hormonal regulations come to the foreground. For example, inhibited aggressive impulses may originally activate the sympathicomedullo-adrenal system, yet this picture becomes masked by the sequence of events in the course of which an increased secretion of corticosteroids produces renal pathology and leads to the development of persistent hypertension. In this instance the primary role of the sympathetic nervous system is lost sight of because of secondary phenomena. The theory of specificity obtains only in regard to the factors which initiate disequilibrations, and not to their secondary results.

The precise relation of neurogenic and hormonal regulations in normal and morbid conditions is still problematical. The studies of Selye, Long, and others are definite steps toward the elucidation of such mechanisms. In his "Adaptation Syndrome," Selye (211) postulated that exposure to any nonspecific noxious stimulus of sufficient intensity results in the liberation of catabolic metabolites in the tissues and the production of the first stage of the syndrome, viz., the "alarm reaction." This stage is divisible into two distinct phases. The first, or "shock phase," is characterized by tachycardia, decrease in muscle tone and body temperature, formation of gastric and intestinal ulcers, hemoconcentration, anuria, edema, hypochlorhydria, leucopenia followed by leucocytosis, acidosis, a transitory hyperglycemia, and finally a decrease in blood sugar and a discharge of epinephrine from the adrenal medulla. Selye postulated that if the damage is not too severe, the catabolic metabolites stimulate the anterior lobe of the pituitary to discharge adrenocorticotropic hormone which, in turn, stimulates the secretion of an excess of adrenal cortical hormones, which help to raise the resistance of the body. This is called the second phase of the alarm reaction, viz., the "counter-shock phase," which is characterized by an enlarged and hyperactive adrenal cortex, rapid involution of the thymus and other lymphatic organs and a reversal of most of the signs characteristic of the shock phase. If the noxious stimulus persists, the countershock phase gives way to the second stage of the general adaptation syndrome, the "stage of resistance." Now most of the morphological lesions observed in the first stage disappear and resistance to the continued stimulus reaches a maximum which is attributed to the cortical hormones. The third and final stage of the syndrome, called the "stage of exhaustion," appears after prolonged exposure to the noxious stimulus and is attributed to a wearing off of the adaptive mechanisms. When this occurs, the lesions characteristic of the alarm reaction reappear, and death ensues. Under special experimental conditions, exposure to nonspecific noxious agents may cause hypertension, nephrosclerosis, myocardial lesions, and arthritis, which Selye attributes to the excessive amounts of anterior pituitary and adrenal cortical hormones produced originally to increase the resistance. For such reasons these derangements are called the "diseases of adaptation." In summary, Selye's concept is that the organism responds to a great variety of stresses with physiological defense mechanisms which are essentially dependent upon the integrity of the adrenal cortex and that excessive activity of this gland is responsible for the diseases of adaptation. The organism is damaged by an excess of its own defensive measures.

Long (142) and his associates added to Selye's observations by showing that the increased secretion of cortical hormone is dependent upon a preliminary activity of the anterior lobe of the pituitary, which in turn is stimulated primarily by epinephrine released from the adrenal medulla. In accordance with Long's observations it would appear that hypothalamic excitation, irrespective of the manner in which it is produced, results in a chain reaction. The first link in this chain is the stimulation of the hypothalamus, which results in stimulation of the sympathetics, followed by increased epinephrine secretion, which in turn induces the secretion of the tropic hormones of the anterior pituitary. The last link in the chain reaction is the stimulation of the hormones of the thyroid and adrenal cortex by the tropic hormones of the anterior pituitary. In other words, the end result of hypothalamic excitations by stress represents the direct effects of the adrenal cortical, thyroid, and other hormones on cellular metabolism.

Recent observations of Sawyer (148, 204) and his co-workers suggest the possibility of a more direct influence of the hypothalamus on the anterior pituitary gland by humoral agents originating in the hypothalamic tissues when they are stimulated by nerve impulses. These investigators demonstrated that the ovulation which occurs in the rabbit within one hour after copulation can be prevented by dibenamine, a drug which inhibits the action of epinephrine if it is administered within three minutes after copulation. It is well established that copulation in the rabbit stimulates the secretion of pituitary gonadotropic hormone and the consequent ovulation only if the sympathetic chain is intact. The intravenous or intracarotid injection of epinephrine is ineffective in producing ovulation, while the direct application of this hormone to the anterior pituitary will produce ovulation. This suggests that through sympathetic stimulation an epinephrine-like substance is produced locally in the hypothalamic tissues and is transported to the pituitary by the blood stream (Fig. II).

These studies give us an idea about the complex interplay of nervous and hormonal mechanisms by which the organism adapts itself to stress and responds in general to external stimuli. It would appear that the neural mechanisms are of primary significance in acute emergency, whereas under chronic stress the ensuing humoral responses come gradually to dominate the picture.

In spite of these secondary complications the above proposed differentiation between the two types of basic responses remains valid: (1) The organism either prepares to meet the stress situation by the mobilization of all its resources which involves a vegetative preparation through the acti-

FIGURE II.

Mechanisms involved in adaptation to stress

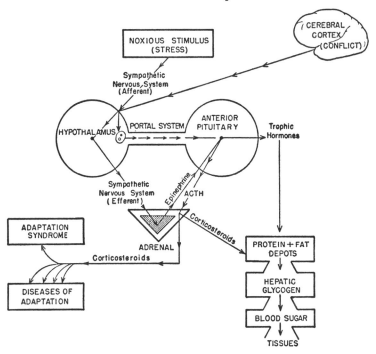

Schematic illustration of the mechanisms involved in the production of the Adaptation Syndrome of Selye as modified in accordance with the observations of Long (140), and Sawyer, *et al.* (204). Stress, be it of organic or psychic origin, stimulates the hypothalamus with a resultant: (1) activation of sympathetic nervous system and the release of epinephrine from the adrenal medulla, and (2) release of a neurohumoral agent from the hypothalamus. As a result, there is a stimulation of the anterior pituitary increasing the secretion of the tropic hormones. (Mirsky.)

vation of the sympathico-medullo-pituitary-adrenal systems; or (2) the organism may retreat from the stress situation by seeking aid from others or by a kind of paralysis of its self-assertive efforts which involve the stimulation of physiological functions regulated by the parasympathetic nervous system. Both responses indicate a disturbance of the autonomic balance provoking counter-regulatory mechanisms which may mask the original disturbance. Psychodynamic studies alone can establish the nature of the initial disturbance and account primarily for the differences by which various individuals respond to the challenges of life. Essentially, this represents the concept of specificity.

Part Two

Emotional Factors in Different Diseases

Introduction to Part Two

THE SYSTEMATIC study of the interrelationship between psychological and physiological factors in chronic disorders of the vegetative systems is of relatively recent origin. Most internists, however, are aware of such a relationship and state unhesitatingly that more than half of their patients suffer from some emotional disturbance which is in large part responsible for their somatic complaints. Examination of the medical literature reveals many references to isolated observations concerning emotional factors in somatic disturbances. Dunbar and Weiss and English have admirably summarized the various observations reported by internists, psychiatrists, and psychoanalysts (71, 75, 242). The vast majority of observers refer to the emotional disturbance as anxiety, a term which is utilized too frequently in describing any kind of emotional tension. Even though the correlation of anxiety with somatic disturbance gives little information as to the specific psychological factors that may be involved, nevertheless such observations have made it apparent that psychiatric care is an important and intrinsic part of the medical management of a patient.

Investigations directed toward the understanding of the specific nature of the emotional factors in the genesis of somatic disturbance and the mechanisms by which they produce such disturbance have received but little attention. A step in that direction was the application of anamnestic interviews by which the pertinent emotional factors are elicited, both in the patient's past and in his present life situations. This procedure, which permits an evaluation of the personality factors and their correlation with particular disease states, has been described in detail by Dunbar (75).

Chapter IX

Emotional Factors in Gastrointestinal Disturbances

THE ALIMENTARY process is the axis of emotional life in early infancy. The child's universe is centered in nutrition, and the strongest emotions, displeasure and gratification, become associated with various aspects of these functions. Even in later life, many phases of the alimentary process remain linked with certain emotional attitudes. Many early reaction patterns are connected with nutrition, such as the secretion of saliva and gastric juice upon exposure to the sight and smell of food. Disgust, which expresses a general rejection of certain objects in the environment, originates in the rejection of certain foods and is associated with reflex phenomena in the esophagus and stomach.

In general, extraverted interest, particularly intense rage or fear, has an inhibitory influence upon the functions of the alimentary tract, upon the secretion of the stomach and bowels as well as upon peristalsis. This inhibition is due to excitation of the sympathetic-adrenal system, as contrasted with excitation of the parasympathetic system, which accelerates gastrointestinal function. The emotional attitudes which normally stimulate the gastrointestinal function are hunger, the sight and smell of food, the desire to be fed, and the less concrete desire to be helped and to relax. In gastrointestinal disorders the harmonious adaptation of the gastrointestinal activity to the general state of the organism is disturbed. An understanding of the psychodynamic background of these disturbances necessitates a detailed review of the normal psychology of the alimentary process.

1. DISTURBANCES OF APPETITE AND EATING

PSYCHOLOGY OF THE NUTRITIONAL PROCESS

No vital function in early life plays such a central role in the emotional household of the organism as does eating. The child experiences the first relief from physical discomfort during nursing; thus the satisfaction of hunger becomes deeply associated with the feeling of well-being and security. The fear of starvation remains the nucleus of insecurity (fear of the future), even though actual starvation is not common in our civilization. In severe melancholia the fear of starvation is often openly expressed by the patient; and it is not uncommon in many psychoneuroses, although the patient may not verbalize it freely. In addition to the sense of security, feeding is deeply associated with the feeling of being loved. For the child, to be fed is equivalent to being loved; in fact, the sense of security associated with satiation is based on this emotional equation (oral receptiveness).

Another emotional attitude of fundamental importance, which becomes linked early in infancy with eating and hunger, is possessiveness, with all its implications, such as greed, jealousy, and envy. To the child, possession is equivalent to bodily (oral) incorporation. The thwarting of this possessive tendency and of the wish to receive leads to aggressive impulses, to take by force that which is not given. Thus, biting becomes the first manifestation of hostility (oral aggression). It is natural that these possessive aggressive impulses centering in oral incorporation should become the sources of the first guilt feelings as soon as the conscience develops. This explains why the psychoanalysis of neurotics suffering from various forms of eating disturbances commonly reveals underlying guilt feelings as the central emotional problem.

Another important emotional connection is that between suckling and pleasurable sensations localized in the mucous membrane of the mouth, lips, and tongue which the infant tries to reproduce by thumb-sucking. These early oral sensations of pleasure may be considered as the forerunners of later genital excitations. This early libidinal role of the mouth survives in adult life in kissing.

These considerations account for the significance of possessiveness, greed, jealousy, envy, and the striving for security in disorders of the alimentary functions. Whenever the emotions described become repressed and thus blocked from expression through voluntary behavior, they create a permanent tension and may exert a chronic disturbing influence, via the vegetative pathways, on different phases of the alimentary process. The asocial, aggressive nature of these emotions makes them particularly apt to create conflict with the environment and consequently leads to their repression. The pleasurable physical sensations connected with the early forms of nutrition (sucking) explain the frequency of emotional disturbances of the nutritional functions when the mature genital functions are inhibited by conflicts. These repressed sexual cravings are expressed regressively in the nutritional process, and their repudiation manifests itself in eating disturbances.

Knowledge of these fundamental psychological facts is necessary for the understanding of the emotional background of neurotic eating disorders. The complexity of psychic life, however, prohibits rigid schematic generalizations; each case must be understood individually. For practical reasons, the various disease entities will be discussed under the usual clinical classifications.

Anorexia nervosa

Periodic or chronic loss of appetite is a common occurrence in psychoneuroses and psychoses, particularly in reactive depressions, during the depressive phase of manic-depressive psychosis, and in schizophrenia. When loss of appetite is the outstanding symptom and when there is no evidence of a major psychosis, the diagnosis "anorexia nervosa" is often made, although this symptom is only one manifestation of a neurotic disturbance of the total personality. In severe anorexia, the patient may lose considerable weight and become seriously emaciated. Women, especially girls after puberty, show this symptom more often than men. A differential diagnosis from Simmonds' disease, where the disturbance of appetite is a secondary result of a pituitary abnormality, is important and not always easy (Richardson—187).

Irrespective of the precise mechanism responsible for the loss of appetite in a particular individual, the decreased intake of food results in marked loss of weight, which may lead to severe emaciation. Concomitant with, or occasionally preceding, the loss of appetite, there may be a cessation of growth and a cessation of menstruation, increased fatigability, loss of axillary hair, disappearance of sexual desire, and other evidences of impaired endocrine function. For such reasons it is difficult to distinguish the effects of starvation on the one hand from the effects of decreased anterior pituitary activity on the other.

The anterior pituitary gland produces the hormones responsible for the stimulation of general body growth, of the gonads, and of the thyroid. In the absence of these hormones there is a cessation of growth and of gonadal and thyroid activity. As a result, the menstrual cycle is interrupted in women and impotence develops in men. Decreased activity of the thyroid results in depressed metabolic activity and in decreased appetite. Since the activity of all cells, including those of the anterior pituitary gland, is dependent in large measure upon the intake of adequate amounts of calories, vitamins, and minerals, relative starvation may produce a diminution in the secretory activity of the anterior pituitary. This has been demonstrated by experiments on animals which were subjected to various degrees of starvation and by the frequent cessation of menstruation in women and impotency in men as a result of malnutrition during periods of famine.

In a study of dwarfism in children, Talbot and his colleagues (232) observed diminished growth as a result of anorexia caused by emotional disturbances. The correction of emotional disturbances, in some instances, was followed by an improvement of the appetite and even by an appreciable increase in the rate of growth. Other children, who did not respond to an improved dietary regime, did respond when growth hormone was administered. These observations indicate that decreased activity of the anterior pituitary gland may occur as a result of decreased caloric intake. This accounts for the difficulties in differentiating a primary insufficiency of the anterior pituitary from that which is secondary to starvation.

Starvation may produce abnormalities in behavior which approximate the characteristic symptoms observed in patients with anorexia nervosa. Illustrative are the studies of Schiele and Brozek (206), who observed during starvation or semi-starvation marked psychological disturbances similar to those observed in patients with anorexia nervosa. It is probable that once anorexia develops in consequence of some psychological disturbance, a vicious circle ensues which may end in a diminished activity of various endocrine glands.

It thus follows that on account of the fine and complex interaction between psychic and endocrine functions, it is futile to try to establish rigidly a "primary" factor. In a 28-year-old woman with severe anorexia nervosa whom I recently observed, amenorrhea developed secondarily to starvation, and the menses returned after recovery. Yet gynecologic examination showed an infantile uterus. Rahman, Richardson, and Ripley (184) found, in a total of twelve cases, four with undeveloped and five with atrophic uterus. Possibly hypogonad types are more inclined to this condition.

The stubborn refusal of the nipple by some infants immediately after birth may perhaps be considered as the earliest prototype of anorexia. We deal in such cases with a resistance of the organism against the new adaptation required by the changed conditions following birth. Some organisms are less flexible in the transition from intrauterine to postnatal existence and manifest a variety of physiological dysfunctions as results of delayed adaptation. Icterus neonatorum, in which the liver continues its intrauterine type of functioning, is another illustration of such a delayed adjustment (Cserna— 53).

Careful psychiatric examination of adults and older children in whom the loss of appetite is not due to pituitary dysfunction will reveal the underlying emotional factors. Even a superficial psychiatric examination may uncover a great variety of neurotic trends. Rahman, Richardson, and Ripley mentioned obsessive, depressive, schizoid features and certain compulsive character trends, such as perfectionism, stubbornness, overconscientiousness, neatness, sensitiveness, and overambitiousness. Richardson (187) and Farquharson (82) also emphasized psychoneurosis as the primary cause. Earlier authors like Gull (107) and Lasègue (135) recognized the etiologic significance of psychological influences. Relevant psychodynamic factors became apparent only after application of the psychoanalytic method.

Psychoanalytic observation shows that unconscious aggressive possessive impulses such as envy and jealousy are the outstanding factors in anorexia. These impulses, if inhibited by the conscience, may lead to severe inhibitions of eating. It is easy to understand that since eating serves as a gratification, the presence of a guilty conscience may disturb the appetite so that the patient will not grant himself the pleasure of satiation. Illustrative of this principle is the fact that fasting is a common form of repentance. Moreover, anorexia may be preceded by an extreme interest in food, even to the extent of bulimia.

Another common psychological factor found in patients with anorexia is an unconscious spite reaction. Through his symptom, the patient behaves like a pouting child who refuses to eat in order to force his parents to pay him special attention and to make them worry. The following case demonstrates the most common emotional factors underlying nervous anorexia:

> In an eight-year-old girl, a severe anorexia developed during the summer vacation. The child refused practically all food, and every meal was the occasion of violent scenes, in which she was forced to swallow a few bites. She lost weight and soon showed clinical evidences of undernourishment. The pediatrician prescribed the usual roborants and completely overlooked the emotional factors. After the psychiatrist had won the child's confidence, it was not difficult to uncover the emotional background of the condition. She had a younger sister, at that time two years old, who was fed by a nurse, usually in the presence of the mother at the same time that the patient ate. The psychiatric interview revealed that the older girl had experienced strong jealousy of her younger sister. This little intruder absorbed all the parents' attention. It became evident that the child's refusal to eat was motivated first by her wish to capture both the nurse's

and the mother's attention and to direct it away from the little sister. By means of her stubborn symptom she succeeded in doing so. The second motive was a guilt reaction. She wanted to receive all the love, to take away everything from her little sister, and she had to do penance for this envy by not eating. The third factor in her anorexia was spite toward the parents, getting revenge for all their attention being given to her younger sister. A few psychiatric interviews in which all these emotions poured out dramatically, and a change in the management of daily routine, promptly eliminated this dangerous symptom. The patient was taken alone by the parents to a restaurant for her meals, which she consumed with her parents. In this way she was given a premium for being the older one, and this helped her tolerate the attention given to her younger sister. Enjoying the advantages of being the older child, she could more readily renounce the privileges of the baby.

The same emotional factors can be discovered in most adults, although they may occur in a more complicated combination. The oral aggressive and receptive tendencies often become erotized and connected with fantasies of sexual practices such as fellatio and cunnilingus. The association of the hunger drive with such ego-alien sexual impulses may also lead to eating difficulties. It is a common fantasy of childhood and early adolescence that impregnation takes place orally. Unconscious pregnancy wishes and fearful rejection of such a desire is among the common emotionally charged fantasies responsible for the eating difficulties of young girls. In other cases coprophilic tendencies may be present.

Other forms of eating inhibitions

Some patients experience no loss of appetite but feel embarrassed and inhibited in attempting to eat in the presence of certain persons. Not uncommonly young girls cannot eat in the presence of men to whom they have an emotional attachment. In such instances the eating disturbance is less generalized, appears only under highly specific conditions, and is not connected with lack of appetite. In spite of being hungry, the patient is inhibited in eating and feels great embarrassment and fear. Unconscious sexual fantasies with aggressive connotation (oral-castrative wishes) usually play an important role in such patients.

The following history is that of a patient treated in the Chicago Institute for Psychoanalysis by Saul.

An attractive twenty-six-year-old girl complained that for the past six years she had not been able to eat in public because of embarrassment, anxiety, nausea, and faintness. This seriously handicapped her social life and her relations with men. She was the oldest of seven children. While the children were still small, the father gave up all efforts to support the family, which sank into poverty. The patient remained overtly cheerful and generous and was soon earning money, but unconsciously she bitterly resented the mother's repeated pregnancies by the lazy, dependent father. Each new child deprived her further of her mother's attentions and increased her burden by bringing another mouth to feed. She expressed her feelings by references to eating and food. For her the most touching expression of love was a gift of food, and when in her dreams she attacked people it was by biting. Her repressed bitterness against her mother resulted in a pervasive sense of guilt. This guilt was attached for specific reasons to eating and sexuality, both of which were consequently inhibited. The eating phobia began when she was taken to dinner by a boy of whom she thought her mother disapproved. She could eat freely only what her mother served her at home, for then she was doing only what her mother urged; then she had her mother's approval and love, and her resentment and guilt were reduced.

In the more generalized anorexias and in the more specific neurotic eating inhibitions, the cause may be uncovered by psychoanalysis. Expert handling is indispensable. Inappropriate psychotherapeutic measures, such as aggressively forcing the patient to eat, may be just as dangerous as artificial feeding. The patient's self-imposed fasting is a means of relieving deep-seated guilt feelings, and the breaking of the symptom without systematic psychotherapy may provoke even more violent self-destructive tendencies, such as attempts at suicide (Richardson—187). The use of drugs or insulin injections can be considered of only symptomatic value.

BULIMIA

Whereas in the patient with anorexia there is a decrease of the appetite because of unconscious emotional factors, in bulimia the appetite is exaggerated. Only rarely do organic factors play a role in bulimia, as in hyperthyroidism, where the appetite is exaggerated as a result of increased metabolism. In psychogenic bulimia, the increased hunger is not the expression of the organism's increased need for food; eating becomes a substitute gratification for frustrated emotional tendencies which have basically nothing to do with the process of nutrition. An abundance of different emotional factors have been described by various psychoanalysts, such as Wulff (259), Schmied (207), Coriat (50), Benedek (27), and others. All are in accord in the belief that the eating disturbance is usually a reaction to emotional frustration. An intense craving for love and aggressive tendencies to devour or to possess form the unconscious basis of the morbidly exaggerated appetite. Unconscious feminine sexual tendencies, pregnancy fantasies, and castrative wishes may also play an important role. The resulting obesity often serves as a defense against the feminine role, which the patient rejects because of its masochistic connotation. The frequency of anorexia nervosa in patients who have suffered from bulimia shows the close relation between the two conditions.

As in the case of other psychogenic disturbances of the appetite, psychotherapy alone can reveal the causes of the disturbance. The aims of the therapy are to bring into consciousness the repressed emotional tensions, thus permitting them to find adequate and acceptable expression in human relationships. Like all psychogenic disturbances of the nutritional process, bulimia is only one symptom of a neurotic disturbance of the total personality.

NERVOUS VOMITING

While in anorexia the incorporative function is inhibited, in patients with nervous vomiting the incorporated food is expelled because of some emotional conflict. The psychoanalytic technique makes it possible, usually, to uncover intensive feelings of guilt, motivated by aggressive, grabbing, incorporating tendencies. The nervous vomiting is the expression of guilt feelings aroused by these wishes. It expresses the tendency to return that which the patient incorporates in his unconscious fantasies. Whereas the patient with anorexia cannot take any food because of guilt feelings, the patient with vomiting has to return food already incorporated on account of the aggressive symbolic significance of the eating act. This mechanism was clearly demonstrated by Levine (137) in a case of chronic vomiting. Bond (33) likewise observed neurotic vomiting in which a guilty conscience was a conspicuous feature. Another factor commonly noted is the rejection of unconscious pregnancy wishes. Illustrative is the history of a patient analyzed by Masserman:

> An intelligent 30-year-old middle-class woman came to analysis with the complaint that for the preceding twelve years she had been subject to menstrual disturbances, food sensitivity, some anorexia, and particularly nausea and vomiting whenever she attempted to have social contacts with men outside her own home. Her illness had forced her to give up many desired recreational and cultural pursuits, and she had almost abandoned all hope of marriage. Psychoanalysis revealed that the patient had been dominated by her possessive, ambitious, and at times tyrannical mother, whose favor she attempted to secure by professed personal devotion, by struggles for scholastic and musical achievement, and later by financial support of the family. This hoped-for security was threatened during late childhood when the mother, jealous of the favoritism shown the patient by her kindly but ineffectual father, began openly to reject her and to favor her three elder sisters. Unfortunately, the patient reacted to the trauma with an even greater fixation of oral dependence

on her mother and an inhibition of all sexual strivings, which she feared might increase her mother's hostility. This inhibition, in line with the patient's infantile fixation on her mother, assumed the form of a disturbance of the nutritional act. Since the mother was the original feeding person, guilt and fear felt toward the mother led to a rejection of the incorporated food. For example, the patient remembered that even at the age of ten she had vomited when a boy brought her food at a party. Concurrently the patient began to fail in her school work, musical studies, and social adjustments and thus acted out her ambivalent attitude toward her mother by thwarting her ambitions. Five years before the analysis, at a time when the patient's guilt and anxiety were increased by the disturbing attentions of a suitor, menstrual disturbances, anorexia, nausea, food sensitivity, and vomiting increased to such an extent that she lost 28 pounds in a few months and was forced to enter a diagnostic clinic. The physical, laboratory, and roentgen findings were normal, and the patient was advised to discontinue all medication and to lead a more active and normal life. Significantly, the patient misinterpreted this advice to mean sexual indulgence and therefore, after obtaining her mother's explicit consent and active co-operation, arranged a liaison with her employer's son. During the seven months that this affair lasted, the patient's symptoms improved, although she remained to some degree frigid and continued to find it difficult to eat in the presence of her lover. When, however, he finally deserted her to get married, her neurotic symptoms reappeared and the patient, giving up all further attempts at heterosexual adjustment, returned to live with her mother. During the first year of the psychoanalytic treatment, the patient with great difficulty acquired some insight into her extreme dependence on her mother and her anxiety-ridden renunciation of oral incorporative, aggressive, and genital desires. The patient later enlarged her extra-familial, social, and heterosexual activities and has since only occasionally experienced her previous symptoms in mild form.

Nervous vomiting, like all neurotic symptoms of the gastro-intestinal tract, must be considered as only one manifestation of a general psychoneurotic disturbance. Its emotional background is similar to that of the neurotic disturbances of eating, and the therapeutic approach is the same. The symptom itself, but not the neurotic disturbance of the total personality, can often be combatted by suggestion or hypnosis, persuasion, rest cures, and sedative medication. Since these therapeutic measures do not eliminate the cause, they are recommended only when the chronic vomiting is so stubborn that immediate help is indicated. Elimination of the symptom alone, however, does not indicate a cure of the neurosis, which, after the vomiting has subsided, may appear in less conspicuous but equally significant symptoms or in some abnormal behavior in life.

2. DISTURBANCES OF THE SWALLOWING ACT

ESOPHAGEAL NEUROSES

Whereas in anorexia and in other eating difficulties the eating act itself is inhibited and in nervous vomiting the incorporated food cannot be retained, in esophageal neuroses the act of swallowing is disturbed. The patient chokes on food and cannot get it down. In some patients a subjective sensation of a foreign body, usually in the upper part of the esophagus, appears independently of eating (globus hystericus).

Kronfeld (134), on the basis of a systematic psychiatric study, distinguished two forms of esophageal neurosis, a sensory hyperalgetic and a reflectory spastic form. The sensory hyperalgetic form is often superimposed on a local disturbance, whereas this does not occur in the spastic form. The emotional basis of the symptoms is an unconscious rejection of incorporation, which is due to aggressive impulses, often of a sexual nature (castration wishes), connected with eating and swallowing. Kronfeld tried to differentiate between the emotional background of anorexia, of esophageal neuroses, and of hysterical vomiting. He compared the esophageal neurotic to the gambler in that both dare to incorporate or take things and expose themselves to an imagined danger. The patient with anorexia simply refuses to eat and in hysterical vomiting the reaction comes only after the crime, symbolized by eating, has already been committed. Kronfeld found that disgust plays an important role in this disturbance. He defines disgust as a combination of temptation and rejection with an ambivalent attitude toward incorporation. Kronfeld's observations still have to be corroborated, although they are in close accord with general psychological data on the eating and swallowing act.

Kronfeld emphasized the need for quick relief in severe esophageal neuroses and therefore he recommended any method which dispels the symptom, such as spasmolytic medication, diathermy, and quickly effective forms of psychotherapy.

As in other disorders, even after the symptom is broken the psychoanalytic approach is indicated for resolving the deeper emotional disturbances of the total personality of which the esophageal symptom is but one manifestation.

CARDIOSPASM

A well-defined disturbance of the swallowing function is known as cardiospasm—a term introduced by von Mikulicz in the nineteenth century. This consists in a contraction of the lower end of the esophagus and leads to a dilatation of the proximal portion. As a result of his psychosomatic investigation of nine patients, Edward Weiss (240) concluded that cardiospasm is a disorder with a somatic predisposition and emotional precipitants in its etiology. He classified cardiospasm superficially as one of the conversion hysterias and assumed that as such it expresses an unconscious symbolic meaning which can be stated as: "I cannot swallow the situation." The symptom appears when a patient finds himself in an emotional impasse in regard to his external situation. In a deeper layer, sexual, hostile, and self-punitive trends are of etiologic significance. Weiss recommends the combined approach of mechanical dilatation and psychotherapy. He emphasized that the treatment of the emotional factors should not be neglected.

He observed a patient who developed a depression immediately after mechanical dilatation.

3. DISTURBANCES OF THE DIGESTIVE FUNCTIONS

GASTRIC NEUROSES

Gastric neuroses display an enormous variety of symptoms based on disturbances of the secretory and motor functions of the stomach and duodenum. It is often difficult to differentiate between neurogenic (central) and organic (local) factors. Many functional gastric symptoms are secondary results of faulty habits of eating. Such habits as incomplete mastication, fast eating, air swallowing, immoderation, and unwise selection of food are frequently the expressions of emotional conflicts, and therefore these disturbances can also be considered as psychogenic. The overtaxing of the stomach by continued unhealthy eating habits may lead to local disturbances (gastritis). The extreme variety and complexity of symptoms makes a rigid differentiation between psychogenic (functional) and local (organic) factors impossible. Nervous disturbances of the stomach may range from slight distress after eating, heartburn, loss of appetite, and regurgitation or eructation of gas to severe gastralgia and intractable vomiting. The physiological basis of these different symptoms is as varied as the symptoms themselves. Hypoacidity seems to appear frequently during depressive states and in connection with fatigue. Chronic hyperacidity with its concomitant symptoms has been observed often to have a psychological background similar to that of peptic ulcer. Comparative clinical studies conducted in the Chicago Institute for Psychoanalysis have shown that in all patients suffering from psychogenic gastric disturbances, a predominant role is played by the repressed help-seeking dependent tendencies. A strong fixation to the early dependent situation of infancy comes in conflict with the adult ego, resulting in hurt pride; and since this dependent attitude is contrary to the wish for independence and self-assertion, it must be re-pressed (Alexander, *et al.*—14). This conflict is most conspicu-ous in cases of peptic ulcer (see pages 102, 103).

That all functional gastric symptoms are influenced by wor-ries, fear, family quarrels, and business reverses is common knowledge in general practice. The extensive experiences of the last war have shown that continuous overexertion and ex-posure to danger are other causative factors. The common denominator in these emotional tensions is an intense longing for rest, security, and help. Accordingly, the improvement of nervous stomach symptoms can be most successfully obtained by rest, change of environment, and relief from emotionally disturbing life situations. The symptoms may resist all forms of drug therapy while the patient is exposed to the stresses of everyday life. When on vacation or in a sanatorium the same patient will show a quick recovery and may be able to dispense with all dietary restrictions without any ill effect. Nevertheless, rest cures or changes of life situations must be considered only as symptomatic measures, because the underlying pathogenic emotional conflicts are not resolved. Most patients have to continue with their professional and social activities and can-not remain permanently segregated from the realities of every-day life. Systematic psychotherapy directed toward the funda-mental problems of the total personality is therefore indicated in all serious cases. The stomach symptoms should be con-sidered only as the indicators of an underlying personality dis-turbance. Undue attention given to the symptoms only sup-ports the neurotic patient's evasion of those emotional prob-lems which underlie the symptoms and thus contributes to the perpetuation of the difficulty. The physician's obligation in such cases is to call the patient's attention to the secondary nature of his physical symptoms and to counteract his flight into organic sickness by urging him to a final showdown—i.e., to undergo psychotherapy, which may make it possible for him to settle his emotional problems. Certain cases in which this strategy is not advisable will be discussed in the chapter on therapy.

PEPTIC ULCERS

The significance of emotional factors in the causation of peptic ulcers is receiving increasingly more emphasis. The more recent studies are only systematic confirmations of isolated observations of a large number of clinicians who for many years have suspected the importance of psychogenic factors in the etiology of this disorder. Von Bergmann (30) and Westphal (246) came to the conclusion that most peptic ulcers may be considered as the "least unpleasant complications" of functional stomach neuroses of long standing.

That a functional disturbance of an organ may in time lead to structural (organic) tissue changes is an etiological fact of primary importance and may be the solution for many etiologic riddles of modern medicine. This was discussed in detail in Chapter 6.

Utilizing the Wolf-Schindler gastroscope, Taylor (234) observed that peptic ulcers may develop in a stomach which is already the seat of diffuse hyperplastic changes in the mucosa (hyperplastic gastritis). However, it is quite probable that such hyperplastic changes are in themselves the results of a functional disturbance (hyperacidity) of long duration. The etiologic problem is, therefore, to establish the origin of this chronic functional disturbance.

Various authors have found that certain types of persons are more inclined to peptic ulcers than others. Alvarez (19) speaks of the efficient, active Jewish businessman, the go-getter type, as being particularly predisposed to them. Hartman (117) characterizes the peptic-ulcer type as the man who is "encountering obstacles that prove to him a trial and handicap, which he must, because of his nature, endeavor to overcome." He claims that Chinese coolies and the Indians of Latin America never have ulcers, and explains this on the basis of the stoic, almost apathetic attitude and the lack of strain and ambition characteristic of these races. According to Hartman, ulcers are a disease of the civilized world and afflict chiefly the striving and ambitious men of western civilization. Draper and Touraine (70) found typical of their patients a rejection of unconscious female tendencies, the same tendencies which, according to psychoanalytic study, are described as oral-receptive or oral-aggressive impulses. The authors complement their psychological studies with anthropologic measurements and try to describe the peptic-ulcer type as characterized psychologically by the presence of masculine protest and rejection of female tendencies, and anatomically as asthenic or longitudinal.

Studies carried out in the Chicago Institute for Psychoanalysis, indicate that gastric symptoms and even peptic ulcers may develop more frequently in one personality type than in others, but the exceptions which we have encountered at an early stage of our research do not encourage us to regard such a generalization as valid. It was not so much a personality type which was found to characterize the patient with an ulcer as it was *a typical conflict situation* which might develop in many different personalities. It was observed that the wish to remain in the dependent infantile situation—to be loved and cared for—was in conflict with the adult ego's pride and aspiration for independence, accomplishment, and self-sufficiency. These two conflicting tendencies reinforce each other in a characteristic way. In overt behavior many peptic-ulcer patients show an exaggerated aggressive, ambitious, independent attitude. They do not like to accept help and burden themselves with all kinds of responsibilities—the type that is so often seen among efficient business executives. This is a reaction to their extreme but unconscious dependence. The continuous struggle and excessive responsibilities reinforce the wish for a dependent relationship. In the depth of his personality, the patient with an ulcer has an unconscious longing for the sheltered existence of the little child. He carefully hides this dependent attitude from himself, however, and represses it so that it cannot find expression in overt behavior, in his personal relations. The repressed longing for love is the unconscious psychological stimulus directly connected with the physiological processes leading finally to ulceration. This longing is the reason for the beneficial effect of rest cures, during which the patient is removed from continuous responsibilities and the daily struggle. After the symptoms become severe or threatening, or after an acute hemorrhage, the patient can give in openly to his wish to withdraw from his responsibilities and no longer needs to repress it. The severe organic illness then justifies such a withdrawal.

Not all patients suffering from peptic ulcer overcompensate for their dependent desires with an outward show of go-getting activity and acceptance of leadership and responsibilities. Many of them are overtly dependent, demanding, and disgruntled. In such persons the dependent tendencies are frustrated not by internal repudiation but by external circumstances. It would appear that the crucial factor in the pathogenesis of ulcer is the frustration of the dependent, help-seeking, and love-demanding desires. When these desires cannot find gratification in human relationships, a chronic emotional stimulus is created which has a specific effect upon the functions of the stomach.

This view, developed in the first gastrointestinal studies, made in the Chicago Institute for Psychoanalysis, has been validated by further research. A considerable number of peptic-ulcer patients analyzed in the Institute showed the prominence of frustrated oral cravings. Van der Heide (237) published two of these cases in detail and another case, quoted briefly on pages 113 and 114, was described by Alexander (13). Kapp, Rosenbaum, and Romano made a careful psychodynamic study of 20 male ulcer patients (129). They found all their patients to be emotionally immature men displaying strong dependent desires which resulted from either rejection or spoiling in childhood. The symptoms of ulcer developed as a reaction to the frustration of dependent cravings. Some of these patients overcompensated for their cravings and appeared to be hard-working and ambitious. The majority, however, were passive and effeminate and expressed their oral desires openly. The authors concluded that "although the conflict situation is similar in all men with peptic ulcer, the resulting personality façade may vary from exaggerated independence to parasitic dependence."

The frustration of a dependent receptive tendency often provokes an aggressive, demanding attitude which is distinguished from the oral-receptive attitude as an oral-aggressive impulse. Recently Szasz et al. (230) have demonstrated the influence of such aggressive incorporating impulses upon stomach functions in a patient in whom the frustration of dependent needs was likewise the determining factor.

Psychosomatic considerations

If the wish to receive, to be loved, to depend on others is rejected by the adult ego or frustrated through external circumstances and consequently cannot find gratification in personal contacts, then often a regressive pathway is used: the wish to be loved becomes converted into the wish to be fed. The repressed longing to receive love and help mobilizes the innervations of the stomach, which since the beginning of the extra-uterine life have been closely associated with the most primitive form of receiving something—namely, with the process of receiving food. The activation of these processes serves as a chronic stimulus to the gastric function. Since this stimulation of the stomach is independent of normal physiological stimuli, such as the need for food, but originates in emotional conflicts entirely independent of the physiological state of hunger, gastric dysfunction may ensue. In such situations *the stomach responds continuously as if food were being*

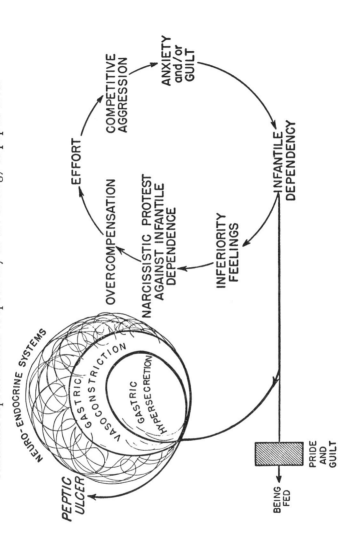

FIGURE III.

Schematic representation of specificity in the etiology of peptic ulcer

taken in or about to be taken in. The greater the rejection of every receptive gratification the greater will be this unconscious "hunger" for love and help. The patient wants food as a symbol of love and help rather than as satiation of a physiological need (Fig. III).

It is suggested that this permanent chronic emotional stimulation of the stomach is similar to that which occurs temporarily during the ingestion of food, with a resultant chronic hypermotility and hypersecretion. The empty stomach is thus constantly exposed to the same physiological stimuli to which it is exposed only periodically, under normal conditions, when it contains or is about to receive food. The symptoms of the "nervous stomach"—viz. epigastric distress, heartburn, and belching—are probably manifestations of this chronic stimulation, which in some cases may lead to ulcer formation (Alexander, *et al.*—14).

The fact that not all patients with gastric neurosis or chronic functional hypersecretion develop ulcers raises the possibility that a constitutional or acquired weakness of the stomach is important in the development of ulceration.

There is growing clinical and experimental evidence for the validity of the psychosomatic view described above. Among internists, Alvarez considers the chronic stimulation of the empty stomach one of the etiological factors of peptic ulcer. In accord are the experiments of Silbermann (212) with sham feeding of dogs. An artificial esophageal fistula was made and the food which the dog swallowed fell to the floor and never reached the stomach; the dog snapped it up again, repeating this procedure sometimes for as long as three-quarters of an hour. Such powerful stimulation of the secretion of the empty stomach, according to Silbermann, leads regularly to ulcer formation. The patient with peptic ulcer is similar to Silbermann's dog in many respects; his stomach is in a state of chronic stimulation, not as a result of eating but as a result of repressed psychological drives to be loved, to receive, or to take aggressively what he does not get freely. Because these tendencies are repressed and excluded from the normal outlet through voluntary behavior, they sustain a permanent tension. The wish to be loved, being closely associated with the wish to be fed, stimulates gastric activity through parasympathetic pathways.

There is much experimental evidence in support of the assumption that one causative factor in ulcer formation may be continuous secretion under the influence of chronic psychological stimuli. The maximum secretion in the stomach occurs during the night in patients with duodenal ulcer (Palmer—178). Winkelstein (252) found high acidity in ulcer patients as a reaction to sham (psychic) feeding and found higher nocturnal acidity in cases of gastric or duodenal ulcer than in normal subjects. These observations show that the stomach of the patient with peptic ulcer is particularly sensitive to nervous stimuli and that continuous secretion is common. Therefore, it would appear that of greater significance than the absolute degree of acidity is the chronic state of excitation of the stomach and the chronic secretion of gastric juice.

The chronic excitation of the stomach induced by emotional tension influences not only the secretory function but the motor functions as well. The specific significance of the latter in the formation of ulcers is not yet clear. Spasm of the pylorus, causing prolonged retention of the acid content of the stomach, may be of etiological significance. The blood supply of the stomach might also be affected. Necheles (175) following Dale and Feldberg's work (54), found that acetylcholine, which under parasympathetic stimuli is liberated in the stomach wall, causes anoxemia in the tissue. Acetylcholine has an influence also on the acid secretion. Necheles also confirmed Winkelstein's findings regarding the higher than normal parasympathetic irritability of ulcer patients.

The clinical findings of the Chicago Institute for Psychoanalysis have received confirmation in the studies of Wolff and

Wolf (258). They studied a patient with a permanent gastric fistula and found hyperemia, hypermotility, and hypersecretion as a reaction to insecurity and to hostile, aggressive feelings when the patient was inhibited, and a return to normal functions when he regained his emotional security. Although these authors considered primarily the conscious mental content and therefore did not reconstruct the psychodynamic situations in detail, the relationship between a longing for security and hyperactivity of the gastric functions can be clearly seen in their observations.

B. Mittelmann and H. G. Wolff (165) subjected the influence of emotions upon gastric activity to an experimental investigation. They induced acute emotional disturbances in both normal individuals and patients suffering from ulcer, gastritis, and duodenitis (26 subjects: 10 ulcer cases, 3 cases of gastritis and duodenitis, 13 normals). They observed in all cases an increase in hydrochloric acid, mucus, and pepsin secretions and an increase in peristalsis; but these were quantitatively more pronounced in the pathological group. The patients with ulcers often reacted with pain, increased bile secretion, and bleeding to the experimentally induced emotional stress which the authors described as anxiety, insecurity, guilt, and frustration. They observed also that in situations which engendered feelings of emotional security and assurance, gastric function was restored to normal.

While the significance of emotional factors in the etiology of peptic ulcer is accepted almost universally today, there is divergence of opinion concerning the specificity of the emotions involved. Those who approach the problem from the clinical side, such as Kapp, Rosenbaum, Romano, Ruesch, and others (129, 199) are impressed by the pronounced oral-receptive trend, manifesting itself either in overt dependence or in its denial.

Mahl, on the basis of an experimental study on dogs, has recently challenged the view that specific emotional conflicts are responsible for increased gastric secretion (144). According to him, the only well-substantiated observation consists in the stimulating influence of chronic fear upon stomach secretion and motility. He maintains that this contradicts Cannon's theory, according to which fear results in sympathetic stimulation which should inhibit and not stimulate gastric activity. Mahl's article is an example of the conceptual confusion which crops up occasionally in the field of psychosomatic research. Many authors without experience and training in psychodynamics almost completely disregard the achievements of the last three decades and try to turn back the clock to a time when the somatic responses were carefully studied but the emotional stimuli which elicit these responses were treated in a most superficial way. They refer to psychological factors in vague terms, such as mental stress, fear, or anxiety, or simply as emotional disturbance in general.

Most of the progress in this field came from the application of the methodological postulate that the psychological chain of events should be studied and described with the same painstaking detail as their somatic sequelae. According to Freud's view, anxiety is internalized fear, a signal for the ego that an unconscious repressed tendency is ready to emerge into consciousness and threaten the ego's integrity. The function of anxiety is the same as that of fear, which is a response to external danger, preparing the ego for meeting the emergency. Anxiety fulfills this function with respect to internal (instinctual) dangers. The ego's defenses against this internal emergency situation are numerous—overcompensation, regression, projection, externalization of anxiety and its displacement to some trivial circumscribed situation (phobias), and many other well-known mechanisms. Which of these various defenses is used depends largely upon the personality structure of the person. The somatic responses to anxiety vary according to the psychological defenses employed. This was discussed in detail on pages 69 and 70. One type of defense against anxiety is treating the internal danger as if it were an external one, preparing to meet it aggressively. This type of defense may produce such symptoms as elevation of blood pressure, increased heart rate, increased muscle tonus, and other somatic signs of sympathetic or voluntary nervous stimulation. Another type of response is regressive. It consists in a retreat to a helpless attitude, running for help and protection. Increased stomach secretion belongs to this type of regressive response to anxiety and fear. It is the manifestation of a regression to the infantile state in which the child turns to mother for help. Since one of the first distresses the child experiences is hunger, which is eliminated by maternal feeding, the wish to be fed becomes the most primitive response to all kinds of emotional stress.

This may suffice to show that at the present stage of our knowledge it is meaningless to speak in general of anxiety as causing somatic symptoms. Anxiety sets in motion different psychological chains, the nature of which is one of the factors determining the type of physiological response which will ensue.[1] Anxiety, the first link in this chain, is not a specific factor. Each person handles anxiety in a manner characteristic for him. This is the meaning of the theory of emotional specificity in the etiology of vegetative diseases.

The final validation of current concepts concerning the role of psychodynamic factors in the etiology of peptic ulcer can come only from studies which are so designed as to permit measurements of gastric activity in men over long periods of time and the correlation of such measurements with concomitant or antecedent emotional factors produced by everyday life situations. An approach to such a procedure has been presented by Mirsky and his colleagues (37, 163, 180), who demonstrated that gastric secretory activity is paralleled by

[1] See also Szasz' discussion of Mahl's paper (223).

the excretion of uropepsin (pepsinogen) in the urine. Their evidence suggests that the rate of uropepsin excretion can serve as an index of the rate of gastric secretion, so that patients with minimal secretion show minimal rates of uropepsin excretion in the urine while those with maximal activity of the stomach show high excretion rates. By means of this technique, the gastric secretory activity of normal subjects and of patients with ulcers and other disorders were measured over various periods of time, up to two years.

A simultaneous record of the significant daily events was kept, such data being obtained either from daily diaries and occasional interviews or from psychoanalytic material. From such studies Mirsky concluded that overt anger, frustration, resentment, and a variety of other dominant emotions of which the subject was aware did not significantly influence the rate of gastric secretion. However, a positive relationship was observed between an augmentation of uropepsin excretion and the mobilization of oral-receptive and incorporative wishes of which the subject was unconscious. Where the individual was conscious of anger or resentment or showed evidences of marked anxiety, analysis of the psychological material revealed clearly that the mobilization of the subject's wish to be taken care of or fear of loss of his dependent relationships was the essential dynamic factor which resulted in an increase in gastric activity.

Therapeutic considerations

In the treatment of peptic ulcer, the first therapeutic consideration must be the treatment of the local condition.

The psychoanalytic theory of the pathogenesis of peptic ulcers has been corroborated in an indirect manner by the recent work of Dragstedt (66) on the treatment of this condition by section of the vagus nerves to the stomach. Although this operation had been tried by others in years past, it was only through Dragstedt's work that vagotomy became a well-understood and useful technique for the therapy of peptic ulcer. The increased and continuous secretion of acid gastric juice typical of patients with duodenal ulcers is mediated by the vagi and is abolished by complete sectioning of this nervous pathway (Dragstedt—64, 65). Incomplete vagotomy is often ineffective in bringing about healing of the lesion. If properly performed, this operation appears to be one of the effective surgical techniques for the treatment of peptic ulcers.

Vagotomy and the other well-established surgical methods do not, however, alter the patient's psychic conflicts, which constitute the primary disturbance in a chain of events leading finally to ulceration in the upper gastrointestinal tract (Alexander—10). Because of this fact, vagotomized patients are prone to develop a number of other more or less serious disturbances. This problem, together with some of the most important sequelae of vagotomy, was studied by Szasz and described by him in a series of publications (226, 227, 228, 229).

Psychotherapy is mainly of preventive value and is aimed at averting recurrences. In most instances there is a variable length of time when functional disturbance is present before the active ulcer develops. Chronic hyperacidity and other stomach symptoms are the first signals that the nervous control of the stomach functions is disturbed. At such times concentration on the local symptoms and neglect of the personality factors is a great error.

Since peptic ulcer is a chronic condition, psychotherapy in combination with medical care of the disorder is indicated. Ulcers usually develop in personalities with a deep-seated neurotic conflict which in itself calls for psychoanalytic treatment. Psychoanalysis offers the best causal approach to the emotional components of ulcer formation. This therapy may vary in duration, since in some instances active psychoanalytic treatment of short duration has proved beneficial.

The following excerpts from a case history may illustrate both the psychodynamic factors involved and the psychotherapeutic aspects of the problem:

A 23-year-old university student had his first hemorrhage from a duodenal ulcer when he was eighteen years old. This was preceded by only a short period of stomach distress. When he came for psychoanalytic treatment five years later he had an active ulcer with typical symptoms and X-ray findings. The patient's most conspicuous personality trait was his extreme casualness, which reflected his marked control over the display of emotion. This was partly due to a fear of appearing soft and weak if he expressed feeling of any kind. As a child the patient had been quiet and obedient, whereas his brother, three years older, had been aggressive and independent. Although the patient was always a good student, he never felt secure among his contemporaries. He tagged along with his brother and the latter's age group and was always under the protection of his brother. He spent much time with his parents, who concentrated their attention on him. When the patient was thirteen the brother died and two years later the father died. These events were of crucial importance in the emotional development. After the death of both older male members of the family, the mother turned to the patient with all her own dependent needs. She consulted him concerning important decisions, forcing him to become a substitute for both the older brother and the father—a task for which he was emotionally unprepared. His casualness and show of imperturbable security were but a defense against insecurity and dependence, which became overwhelming under his mother's exaggerated expectations. This conflict showed itself conspicuously in his relationship to women; he did not allow himself to become emotionally involved, had only casual sexual relationships, and terminated each affair as soon as the woman showed some personal interest in him. He suffered from premature ejaculation. At the beginning of his treatment, this patient was not the least aware of his deep, dependent attachment, directed at first toward his mother, and later toward his father and older brother. He was conscious only of his defense against these feelings. To become emotionally attached to a woman or a man meant weakness to him, and he therefore persuaded himself and others of his indifference and emotional aloofness. These dependent longings became gradually conscious during treatment. At first he recognized his resentment against the mother who, instead of giving him support, leaned on him. In an early dream during treatment he was riding a bicycle with his mother; he was at the handlebars but lost control, and both of them fell. The mother was hurt and probably died. Here the assumption of the role of leadership in relation to the mother is clearly expressed. In the course of the analysis, not only the repudiation of the responsibility but also his deep-seated longing for dependence came to the surface. The latter consisted in an infantile attachment to the mother blended with a passive homosexual attitude which was originally directed toward the father and older brother. The homosexual longings were overcompensated for by aggressive competition, but as soon as these defenses were penetrated the repressed dependence showed itself openly in his transference attitude. At this time he became conscious of his hidden dependent attitude toward his mother, so that he was able to combat this feeling on a conscious level instead of repressing and denying it by assuming a façade of casualness. He succeeded gradually in renouncing more and more of his excessive dependency and in accepting a more mature attitude. With these internal developments a profound change took place in his relationship to women. He fell in love with a young woman, and for the first time in his life a prolonged happy sexual affair ensued. He later married her. At the same time his stomach complaints diminished and he was able to live on a normal diet with only occasional mild distress.

The treatment of this patient lasted for ten months, during which he was seen thirty-six times. His condition was followed up for the next three years and occasionally he was seen in therapeutic interviews. He had two mild relapses, the first one shortly after his marriage, when he accepted a very strenuous assignment abroad and had to live on an unsuitable diet. The second relapse occurred a few weeks before his wife delivered her first child and at a time when his mother was contemplating marriage. He became tense and some marital difficulties began to develop. To his irritable and demanding attitude his wife responded with an emotional withdrawal. The residues of his former dependent attachment to his mother, which he had transferred to some degree to his wife, were mobilized by these two coincidental events. The baby threatened his dependence on his wife and his mother's impending marriage revived the old attachment to her.

In a brief series of consultations he worked through this flare-up of the old conflict and regained his former emotional and physical equilibrium. The marital difficulties, which were partially due to his wife's reaction to her first child, also improved gradually. When he was last seen the patient's complaints were limited to an occasional mild stomach distress upon awakening. He was on a normal diet and his only medication was an evening dose of atropine.

In this case the personality change achieved by psychoanalytic therapy was quite pronounced. The stomach condition has improved markedly; the pathological process has been obviously checked, but the vulnerability of the seriously damaged organ may not be completely reversible.

Specific Dynamic Patterns in Gastric Hyperfunction

I

Frustration of oral-receptive longings ⟶ oral-aggressive response ⟶ guilt ⟶ anxiety ⟶ overcompensation for oral aggression and dependence by actual successful accomplishments in responsible activities ⟶ increased unconscious oral-dependent cravings as reaction to excessive effort and concentration ⟶ gastric hypersecretion.

II

Prolonged frustration of oral-receptive longings ⟶ repression of these wishes ⟶ gastric hypersecretion.

4. DISTURBANCES OF THE ELIMINATIVE FUNCTIONS

PSYCHOLOGY OF THE EXCREMENTAL FUNCTIONS

Next to ingestion of food, the excremental functions play the most important role in the emotional life of the infant. As in food intake, the excremental functions become associated with certain typical emotional attitudes in early life. Before the advent of psychoanalysis, the psychological aspects of these functions were wholly unknown or neglected. These subjects, particularly their psychology, were excluded not only from polite conversation but from scientific investigation and even from medical consideration. A large body of psychoanalytic literature on this subject has accumulated covering data carefully observed over a period of thirty years.

While the desire for security and the wish to receive or to take by force what is not given freely, to be loved, to lean on someone, are most closely associated with the incorporative aspects of nutrition, the eliminative act becomes connected in early life with the emotions of possessiveness, pride in accomplishment, the tendency to give and to retain. Certain types of hostile impulses (attacking, soiling) are also associated with these functions.

The pleasurable sensations connected with suckling are thwarted very early in life. The child reacts to weaning from the nipple with thumb-sucking, which the parents usually try to check. The child then discovers that a similar pleasurable sensation can be procured at the other end of the alimentary tract by the retention of feces. Here too, a solid body stimulates the mucous membrane of a tubular organ. It is more difficult for the adult to interfere with this type of pleasure, and the child therefore develops a sense of independence which soon becomes associated with the excremental act. He loses his sovereignty over his excremental functions, however, during the period of toilet training, when adults try to teach him to move his bowels at regular intervals. For the child this means compliance with the wishes of the adults; he is urged to part with his excrement not when he wishes but when the adults consider it appropriate. In exchange he receives praise, love, and sometimes material goods, such as a piece of candy. In some such manner the excrement becomes associated with the concept of possession. This explains its close relation to money, which is one of the best-established facts uncovered by psychoanalysis. Every excremental act is evaluated by the child as a kind of donation to the adults, an attitude often reinforced by the mother's great interest in the child's excrement. (The German expression for the bowel movement of the child, "Bescherung" means gift.)

The child's earliest attitude toward his excreta is a coprophilic one. The excrement is a valuable possession, a source of pleasure and something which can be exchanged for other goods. This coprophilic attitude, however, is inhibited by educational procedures and changed into its opposite, disgust and depreciation, which becomes the basis of the sadistic aggressive-and-soiling connotation of the excremental act. The excrement becomes a soiling weapon, and the act itself assumes a deprecatory significance. This is exemplified by the little street urchin who defiantly shows his hind parts and often accompanies this gesture with some kind of aggressive invitation. In later life all these emotional connections, to a greater or lesser degree, disappear from the conscious personality, but remain deeply rooted in the emotional life, so that they may appear in neurotic symptoms of mentally disturbed patients and even in the dreams of normal adults.

These early phases of emotional development provide the explanation for the fact that the excremental function becomes connected with the feeling of accomplishment, with giving or attacking, and also that the excrement becomes the symbol of possession. For the understanding of the psycho-

logical background of disturbances of the excremental functions, both psychogenic diarrhea and psychogenic constipation, the knowledge of this emotional development is of
fundamental significance.

CHRONIC DIARRHEA, SPASTIC COLITIS, MUCOUS COLITIS

It is an open question whether these different forms of
intestinal disturbance are different phases or different manifestations of the same basic condition. There is no doubt that
emotional factors play a role in all of these disturbances.
Sometimes the emotional factors may have a primary etiologic
significance. In other cases they only aggravate an existing
local disorder.

Chronic diarrhea can be a symptom of both organic and
neurotic disturbances which may be present simultaneously,
and it is not always possible to distinguish clearly between neurogenic and local pathologic factors. Simple chronic diarrhea
is often the bodily expression of a psychoneurotic condition,
and is the predominating symptom in certain cases. Daily
evacuation of small or large quantities of liquid stool may
take place more or less frequently with or without tenesmus.
In some cases, twenty to thirty evacuations may occur in one
day without any evidence of organic change. Many patients
react to diarrhea with worry and anxiety: they expect it fearfully and their concern about it often becomes the central
issue of their daily life. Many patients name dietary transgres-
sions as the precipitating factors, but others notice some
connection with emotional tension.

Mucous colitis has been considered a neurosis for a long
time. White, Cobb, and Jones (247) concluded that mucous
colitis is a disorder of the physiologic function of the colon
which is brought about through the excessive activity of the
parasympathetic nervous system, which in turn could be attributed to emotional tension in 92 per cent of their cases.
They described certain personality trends which seem to be

characteristic. Their psychologic findings coincided to a great extent with those of the Chicago Institute for Psychoanalysis on various forms of colitis (Wilson—251). Overconscientiousness, dependence, sensitivity, anxiety, guilt, and resentment are the emotional trends most commonly found in patients suffering from mucous colitis.

Psychoanalytic studies of patients suffering from chronic diarrhea and from spastic and mucous colitis reveal a typical conflict centering in their strong demanding (oral-aggressive) and receptive wishes. These patients try to compensate for these dependent wishes by activity and the urge to give by substituting attacks of diarrhea for real accomplishment and giving. They want to give compensation for all those things which they want to receive or take away from others. This often takes the form of worry about certain duties and obligations, the need to give money or support others, the urge to exert effort and to work. For such reasons the patient is often described as being overconscientious. At the same time, however, he has a violent reluctance to exert himself, to engage in systematic strenuous work, and to fulfill those obligations to which he feels compelled emotionally. The repressed psychological factor related to the symptom is the powerful need to give, to make restitution. The patient may become dependent on others but feels he should do something to make compensation for all that he receives. Instead of real accomplishment, however, he satisfies his conscience with this infantile form of gift—the intestinal content.

In this respect the patient shows a conspicuous difference from the patient with peptic ulcer, who also overcompensates for his passive and receptive tendencies, but does so by real exertion, by his efficiency and aggressive, independent behavior in life. The diarrhea patient overcompensates for passivity only through the unconscious symbolism of the excremental act, an emotional substitute for real performance, gifts, and obligations toward others. The physiological basis of such emotionally conditioned chronic diarrhea is obviously the chronic excitation of peristaltic bowel activity induced by excessive stimulation of parasympathetic pathways. The emotional tendencies to give and to accomplish, which arise as compensation for strong receptive or taking tendencies, if repressed and thus excluded from voluntary expression, seem to have a specific influence on the functions of the bowel. Hostile impulses contribute to the development of guilt feelings and the wish to make restitution. In addition, hostile impulses may have a direct effect on the intestinal symptoms.

A male patient, aged 48, was suffering from chronic diarrhea. This condition had lasted for eight or nine years with some remissions. At the beginning, some mucus was found; later the patient had several watery stools a day, felt fatigued, and was extremely concerned with his bowel movements. Every day he dreaded the diarrhea, although it was not painful, and anticipated it fearfully. After evacuation he felt exhausted, unable to work or to concentrate. He could seldom engage in continuous business activity and had to take frequent vacations, during which his condition would improve considerably. He lived on a strict diet, avoiding alcoholic drinks, roughage, fats, and all heavy meals. Various drugs were ineffective. Like many patients with colitis, he reacted favorably to psychoanalytic treatment shortly after its beginning; the diarrhea disappeared almost immediately and returned only occasionally. It was obvious that the emotional relief which the treatment gave him was of immediate symptomatic benefit. During the treatment the conflict between a strong sense of obligation toward his family and others and a strong passive, dependent attitude became apparent.

The patient had married into a wealthy family which made him feel he was an intruder, but at the same time made it possible for the couple to live according to the standards to which the wife had been accustomed. They also helped him financially to develop his business. From the time he married, the patient's life was a desperate struggle to make good through his own effort. He pursued his business activities spasmodically, indulged in long vacations and at the same time revolted internally against all the exertion, wanting to live a leisurely life of travel, sports, and the reading of fine books—the life of a gentleman. The analytic sessions clearly brought out this conflict, which had not been fully conscious and verbalized before. The patient reacted with diarrhea whenever the urge for accomplishment, work, and fulfilling obligations became very intense in him, but at the same time the resistance to carrying out these things in reality became equally potent. It seems that the diarrhea was an infantile method of solution for this conflict. For his unconscious mind, bowel movements still meant accomplishment and giving. This explains why after every evacuation he emphasized the feeling that he was totally cleaned out and exhausted. The bowel movements not only substituted for real exertion in life but also gave him an excuse for relaxation and being taken care of.

An interesting feature of this case is that about eleven years before the diarrhea developed the patient was operated on for gastric ulcer. The ulcer symptoms started when as a student he was making strenuous efforts to satisfy an ambitious mother. The patient concentrated completely on making a career. After the ulcer symptoms had lasted for five years the patient was operated on because of a perforation at a period when he was extremely active, concentrating doggedly on his studies. The diarrhea, which started eleven years later, developed after the marriage through which he became wealthy and to some degree dependent on his wife's family.

This case demonstrates that it is erroneous to assume that certain psychogenic disturbances develop only in certain personality types. The organic condition can be correlated with certain psychodynamic situations but not with personality types. It is obvious that here the same personality was exposed to different conflict situations. While a student he worked hard and reacted to this with a strong longing for dependence, which he did not admit to himself. Then the peptic ulcer developed. When he was living in affluence but in emotional dependence on the wealthy family of his wife, there developed a strong sense of obligation to work hard, which he fulfilled only halfheartedly, interrupting his work as often as possible. At this time chronic diarrhea appeared. His diarrhea was a means of relieving this sense of obligation by a primitive form of giving and accomplishment.

Although dietary measures may be of benefit in these cases, the primary aim of therapy must be directed toward elimination of the emotional disturbance. As with all organ neuroses, rest cures and sedative medication may alleviate symptoms, but the basic condition can be remedied only by psychotherapy.

In cases of chronic diarrhea and spastic and mucous colitis, the value of the psychotherapeutic approach has been demonstrated by the systematic studies of the Chicago Institute for Psychoanalysis, which revealed that most patients can dispense with further dietary restrictions after successful psychoanalytic therapy.

ULCERATIVE COLITIS

Since the publications of Murray (173, 174) and of Sullivan and his co-workers (222, 41), the significance of emotional factors for the precipitation and clinical course of ulcerative colitis has been widely recognized. More or less systematic studies of a series of cases have been published by Wittkower (254), Daniels (56, 57, 58), Lindemann (141), Groen (106), and Ross (196); Jackson (123) and Rosenbaum and Kapp (195) have reported isolated case studies; and Melitta Sperling (218) has presented psychoanalytic observations based on the treatment of two children with ulcerative colitis. But in spite of the considerable clinical material, the specific psychodynamic factors characterizing these patients has not been clearly elucidated.[1] The precise physiological mechanisms responsible for pathological processes in the mucous membrane of the large bowel are also controversial.

The careful student of the literature, however, cannot help being impressed by the consistent recurrence of certain observations and psychodynamic formulations. Murray, who

---

[1] It must be noted that except for a single case described by Daniels, no adult patient has been subjected to what may be considered a thoroughgoing psychoanalysis.

reported the first systematic study of twelve cases, found that conflicts centering in marital relationships were the most common psychologic factors in the precipitation of the illness. Conflicts about sexual relations, and more specifically about pregnancy and abortion, appear in a large number of cases. Sullivan, whose careful observations greatly influenced later research, emphasized that no specific type of precipitating situation is present, ". . . but in each case . . . the patient had been involved in an adjustment situation which was difficult for him as an individual and to which he had responded with tension and anxiety."

It has been emphasized by some investigators that the patient with ulcerative colitis differs from patients suffering from other forms of colitis, with respect to the narcissistic organization of their personalities. In addition Daniels noted the presence of a self-destructive suicidal component. Lindemann was impressed by the impoverished human interrelationships of these patients. Groen attempted to describe a typical personality profile characteristic of these patients on the basis of his study of six cases, but the size of his sample does not make such generalizations valid. Moreover, only the manifest character traits were considered and not the dynamic factors. Melitta Sperling attempted to reconstruct a conflict situation typical of these patients and concluded that ulcerative colitis represents the "somatic dramatization" of melancholia. She postulated that the organism is attacked by the aggressive hostile incorporated object and tries to free itself by immediate anal discharge. Most authors make some reference to the regressive pregenital emotional organization of these patients, to their prevailing anal characteristics, their unusually strong dependence upon the mother combined with ambivalence, which results in repressed sadistic hostile impulses.

Studies at the Chicago Institute for Psychoanalysis reveal the prevalence of those emotional factors which from early life are associated with the excremental and alimentary functions. In this respect, ulcerative colitis patients closely resemble the patients suffering from other forms of diarrhea. Whether psychodynamic differentiation is possible between this and other forms of colitis can only be answered after further detailed studies of unconscious material and personality structure. The fact that the integrative capacity of the ego of many patients with ulcerative colitis is relatively weak and that consequently there is a tendency toward projection and psychotic episodes may prove of some significance.

The presenting psychological material which recurs conspicuously in these patients is best understood on the basis of the general psychodynamics of the excremental function. Two emotional factors are conspicuous in the precipitation of the disease and in the provocation of relapses. One is the frustrated tendency to carry out an obligation, be it biological, moral, or material, and the second is a frustrated ambition to accomplish something which requires the concentrated expenditure of energy. In women, this most frequently consists in conflicts about giving birth to a child or of living up to maternal responsibilities. In some instances, the pressure of financial obligation plays a conspicuous role. Portis quotes the history of a patient which demonstrates this type of emotional dynamics.[1]

A young woman married for six months began suffering from early ulcerative colitis. Under medical management . . . the bowel had become entirely quiescent—no blood, normally formed stools, and a feeling of well-being. After three months of medical management she complained of a precipitous recurrence of her diarrhea on the preceding Sunday morning. Careful interrogation revealed that she had had no undue excitement on the previous Saturday evening. She had eaten at home on Saturday and Sunday, followed her diet religiously and taken her medicine as directed. About one hour after breakfast, while

[1] S. Portis: "Newer Concepts of the Etiology and Management of Idiopathic Ulcerative Colitis," *J.A.M.A.* 139: 208, 1949.

she was working around the home, diarrhea appeared. When further questioned on the situations of that Sunday morning when she was at home with her husband, at first she denied any unusual happening, but further prying revealed that her husband asked her, facetiously or otherwise, "What about the $400 I loaned you when we first got married to buy your trousseau? When am I going to get it back?" She didn't have the $400. She felt distinctly disturbed, regressed into a childhood pattern and got diarrhea. When the analyst pointed out to her the association with the money and her inability to give it back except with bowel movements, the condition immediately cleared up— mind you, with no change in diet or medical management. This patient subsequently went through an entire pregnancy without further recurrence of symptoms.

Financial obligations which are beyond the patient's means are a common factor in some forms of diarrhea. This was recognized by Abraham (4), who described the emotional correlation between bowel movement and the spending of money. Consequently, it is possible that financial involvement is not a specific stimulus to the development of ulcerative colitis but serves as a general stimulus to the activation of bowel functions, which, in an already diseased organ, may precipitate an attack. The question as to whether the emotional conflicts typical of ulcerative colitis differ from those of other forms of diarrhea remains an open one. What seems to be certain is that all forms of anal-regressive emotional stimuli have a specific affinity to the function of the colon.

The first symptom of ulcerative colitis frequently appears when the patient is facing a life situation which requires some outstanding accomplishment for which the patient feels unprepared. The psychodynamic implication can be best understood on the basis of the infant's emotional evaluation of the excremental act, which signified giving up a cherished possession on the one hand and an accomplishment on the other. In persons with this type of emotional fixation, whenever the urge or necessity to give arises in later life or the realization of an ambition on some adult level is blocked by neurotic inhibitions, a regression to the anal form of giving or accomplishment may take place. It should be emphasized, however, that anal regression of this type is extremely common in all kinds of diarrhea and in psychoneurotics who do not display any somatic symptoms. Some specific local somatic factor may be responsible for the fact that in some patients anal regression produces ulceration in the bowels. It is quite probable that the specific factors will turn out to be not psychological but the peculiarity of the physiological mechanisms initiated by the emotional stimuli.

Although it may be premature to discard the possibility that the psychodynamic background in ulcerative colitis has a specific feature not found in other forms of bowel disturbance with diarrhea, one must warn against the readiness of certain authors to interpret psychological findings in these and other organic diseases always as causative in nature. Organic symptoms such as diarrhea give opportunity for patients to utilize the symptom for their psychoneurotic needs. Patients suffering from diarrhea, irrespective of its cause, often exploit this symptom emotionally for a symbolic expression of being exhausted, completely "cleaned out," and may use this symptom as a symbolic expression of castration. Melitta Sperling's psychodynamic reconstructions may be secondary symbolic elaborations of the existing diarrhea. The fantasy of eliminating an incorporated dangerous, bad mother is probably a secondary utilization of the symptom for unconscious emotional needs rather than the cause of it. The causative psychodynamic factors are probably much more elementary and less conceptual in nature. The excremental act as an expression of giving a gift or carrying out an obligation, or as an accomplishment— these and the later aggressive hostile connotation of defecation are the fundamental psychodynamic factors which have a causal relationship to functional bowel disturbances.

Concerning the physiological mechanisms, a publication by Portis (181) deserves special mention. He follows the original suggestions of Murray and more explicitly those of Sullivan that the disease has a neurogenic component. Certain emotional conflict situations transmit a nervous excitation through the vegetative centers via the parasympathetic pathways to the colon. Sullivan assumed that the digestive power of the fast-moving liquid content of the small intestines is higher than normal or the natural protective power of the mucous membrane of the colon may be low. At any rate, surface digestion of the mucosa of the colon occurs and prepares the way for bacterial invasion. In this way acute ulceration results. Portis, in general, accepts this theory. It is his view, which is based on the experimental work of Karl Meyer, *et al.* (155, 156), that through parasympathetic influences, lysozyme, a mucolitic enzyme, increases and deprives the mucosa of its protective mucin so that it becomes more vulnerable to the tryptic enzyme present in the intestinal content. According to Portis, the initial localization of the ulceration is always in that part of the large bowel which is under the nervous control of the sacropelvic portion of the parasympathetic system. Thus localization of the symptoms in early cases is important and confirms the psychiatric observation that the psychological stimuli involved pertain to the excremental act.

The relative significance of inherent constitutional factors concerning the vulnerability of the mucosa of the colon—i.e., disturbed physiological mechanisms based on previous local disease of the colon—invasion by microorganisms, and specific emotional conflict situations cannot be evaluated at the present state of our knowledge. It is important to consider the fact that the same type of conflict situation is found in compulsion neurotics and patients suffering from paranoid symptoms who may not have any significant bowel disturbance or any somatic symptoms. It is probable that some local somatic factor such as that suggested by Murray, Sullivan, and Portis may determine whether the regressive evasion of a conflictful life situation in one patient produces symptoms entirely on the psychological level (obsessive-compulsive symptoms, compulsive character traits, or paranoid delusions) and in other cases leads to some organic bowel disturbance.

Specific Dynamic Pattern in Diarrhea

Frustration of oral dependent longings ——> oral-aggressive responses ——> guilt ——> anxiety ——> overcompensation for oral aggression by the urge to give (restitution) and to accomplish ——> inhibition and failure of the effort to give and accomplish ——> *diarrhea.*

CHRONIC PSYCHOGENIC CONSTIPATION

Chronic psychogenic constipation must be distinguished from the constipation observed in spastic colitis. In some cases constipation is the only gastrointestinal symptom. Although it may be a manifestation of any of various organic conditions, it is usually due to some psychological factor. The psychogenic findings in cases of chronic constipation are typical and constant: a pessimistic, defeatist attitude, a distrust or lack of confidence in others, the feeling of being rejected and not loved, are often observed in these patients. In an exaggerated form this attitude is observed in paranoia as well as in severe melancholia. Chronically constipated patients have a trace of both attitudes: the distrust of paranoia and the pessimism and defeatism of melancholia. In accord are the studies of Alexander and Menninger (15), who found that a statistically significant group of patients suffering from persecutory delusions also suffered from severe constipation; melancholic patients also show a marked tendency toward constipation.

The emotional undertone of chronic psychogenic constipation may be described as follows: "I cannot expect anything from anybody, and therefore I do not need to give anything. I must hold on to what I have." This possessive attitude, which is the outcome of the feeling of rejection and distrust, then manifests itself organically in the constipation. The excrement is retained as if it were a valuable possession; this attitude is in accordance with the early coprophilic attitude of the child. Another psychologic finding, which is usually more repressed, is an unconscious aggressive and depreciatory attitude toward others, which in turn may be a reaction to the general feeling of being rejected. This attitude is deeply repressed and inhibited; the inhibition extends over the excretory function, which for the unconscious life has the significance of a hostile attack and soiling.

The following case is illustrative:

A young woman, married for two years, had suffered from chronic constipation since her marriage. Daily enemas were used. Repeated physical examinations were always negative. Before the analysis, the patient was observed for several days in a hospital for internal disturbances, and the report was: "Organic examination negative, nervous constipation." Analysis revealed the following situation:

The patient entered marriage expecting great love and tenderness, but her husband was an artist whose chief interest was his profession. He was entirely blind to the emotional needs of a young woman and continued a kind of bachelor existence after his marriage. The young wife had a great conscious longing for a child, but her husband refused it because of financial considerations and because he wanted to devote himself entirely to his art. For a long time the analysis did not give any specific clue to the symptom, although it appeared obvious that it was somehow connected with the woman's emotional reaction to her husband's behavior. In order to obtain a personal impression of the husband, the therapist asked to see him. This interview corroborated the patient's description. He appeared to be an interesting but entirely self-centered young man who was naïve and inexperienced in all female affairs. He was unable to understand the therapist's statement that his wife was basically dissatisfied with her marriage, although she herself did not want to recognize this, and repressed her dissatisfaction as much as possible. She lived with the illusion of being happily married and never expressed any direct complaint against her husband. When she said anything which sounded like an accusation against her husband, she did so in a humorous way, as if it were a trifle not worth mentioning. To explain to the husband his lack of attention to his wife, the therapist used an example which the patient had told the therapist characterizing their marital life: that since the first day of their marriage the husband had never brought her any small sign of attention—flowers or anything else. The interview made a deep impression on the husband, and he left the office with a guilty conscience. The next day the patient reported that for the first time in two years she had had a spontaneous bowel movement before she took her daily enema. Seemingly, without any connection, she also reported that her husband had brought home a beautiful bouquet of flowers for the first time in their married life. The cathartic influence of these flowers was amusing and gave us the first clue to the psychic background of the symptom. This woman had used an infantile way of expressing spite toward her husband as an answer to his loveless behavior. The constipation of the patient expressed an infantile reaction which she did not want to admit to herself and which she had never shown openly. She expressed her resentment against the loveless attitude of her husband in this concealed and infantile way. Indeed, the first time her husband was generous, she also became generous and gave up her obstinacy, i.e., her constipation, which had started a few weeks after her marriage. Further analysis proved that upon this early infantile nucleus of spite another motivation was superimposed —namely, the wish to become pregnant. The constipation was a reaction to her husband's refusal to have a child. The unconscious identification of child and excrement was the basis of this reaction. The constipated patient surrendered in a relatively short analysis to this insight. She could no longer deceive herself about her deep dissatisfaction with her husband's behavior, but since her resentment became conscious there was no need to express it in this concealed way. She now had to face her marital problem consciously. After the analysis was finished, the constipation did not return. The fact that a few years after the cure she had a child probably contributed to the permanency of this therapeutic success.

An interesting confirmation of these concepts came from the previously mentioned clinical study of the relationship between persecutory delusion and chronic psychogenic constipation. Alexander and Menninger found in a statistical study that in 100 cases of persecutory delusion 72 per cent suffered from constipation, in contrast with 100 control cases, where the incidence of constipation was only 26 per cent. On the basis of psychodynamic material it was concluded that the frequent constipation of patients suffering from persecutory delusions is mainly conditioned by their conflict over anal-sadistic tendencies which are denied and projected. They found that patients suffering from depressions are also inclined toward constipation. This correlation is most probably due to their emotional attitude. They feel rejected and do not expect to receive from others. Hence their tendency to hold on to their possession and to the most primitive form of possession, the intestinal content.

Chronic constipation is often considered a trivial symptom, and in most cases a symptomatic approach, by dietary measures, laxative medication, enemas, or massage, suffices for all practical purposes. On the other hand, this symptom may be the manifestation of a deep-seated emotional disturbance, and psychoanalysis, as well as briefer psychotherapeutic procedures aiming at the uncovering of unconscious conflicts, often achieves excellent results. Many patients who for years were accustomed to using laxatives have been able to dispense with all further use of drugs as a result of psychotherapy. Of course, constipation is only one, and often not even the most significant, manifestation of a disturbance of the patient's emotional outlook toward life and toward others, and in such cases psychotherapy must be directed toward a reorientation of the total personality.

Chapter X

Emotional Factors in Respiratory Disturbances

THE INFLUENCE of emotion upon the respiratory function is well known from everyday life. Sudden cessation of breathing in anxiety is referred to in such expressions as "breathtaking" or "it took my breath away." Sighing is a common expression of despair. Crying is another complex expressive phenomenon in which the expiratory phase of respiration is involved. And above all, respiration is an important component in speaking.

Because of this close correlation between emotional tensions and the respiratory functions it is probable that in most diseases of the respiratory organs psychological factors play an important role. There are isolated observations in the literature describing emotional influences in the precipitation of tuberculosis (Coleman, Benjamin—29). Systematic studies in this field, however, have been restricted, up to date, to the study of bronchial asthma.

BRONCHIAL ASTHMA

In asthma, as in other disturbances of vegetative functions, the emotional factor is based on normal physiological responses to emotional stimuli. The symptoms are exaggerated and chronic responses to underlying emotions; the exaggerated and chronic nature of the response is basically due to the fact that the emotional stimulus is unconscious because it is unacceptable to the conscious personality. The history of medical knowledge concerning the emotional components in asthma is a long one. Until the allergic phenomena were discovered, asthma was considered primarily a nervous disease and is referred to in older medical textbooks as "asthma nervosa." With the advent of modern immunology, in which the phenomenon of anaphylaxis was a cornerstone, attention became focused on the allergic component, and the older view of asthma as a nervous disease came to be considered obsolete. More recently, in the era of psychosomatic orientation, the emotional etiology of asthma was revived. Isolated clinical observations concerning a great variety of precipitating factors in asthma attacks are numerous. These were reviewed in a monograph by French and Alexander (89) and earlier by Dunbar (74) and by Wittkower (253). A great variety of emotional factors have been mentioned by different observers; they include almost any sudden intensive emotional stimulus—sexual excitation, anxiety, jealousy, and rage. The view of asthma cases here presented is based primarily on the studies in the Chicago Institute for Psychoanalysis, described in detail in the above-mentioned monograph. In these studies it was found that behind this confusing variety of emotional factors, a central psychological constellation can be discerned.

Only the fundamental psychodynamic factors in their relation to allergy will be discussed here. The nuclear psychodynamic factor is a conflict centering in an excessive unresolved dependence upon the mother. As a defense against this infantile fixation all kinds of personality traits may develop. Accordingly, we find among persons suffering from asthma many types of personalities: aggressive, ambitious, argumentative persons, daredevils, and also hypersensitive, aesthetic types. Some asthmatics are compulsive characters, while others are more of a hysterical nature. It would be futile to define a characteristic profile; no such profile exists. The repressed dependence upon the mother is, however, a constant feature around which different types of character defenses may develop. This dependence seems to have a different connotation from that found in gastric neuroses and peptic ulcers. Its content is not so much the oral wish to be fed; it is more the wish to be protected—to be encompassed by the mother or the maternal image. In contrast to the ulcer cases, fantasies of eating and food are not prominent. Instead, there is a high frequency of intrauterine fantasies which appear in the form of water symbolism or entering caves, closed places, etc. (French, Alexander, *et al.*—89). Everything which threatens to separate the patient from the protective mother or her substitute is apt to precipitate an asthmatic attack. In children, the birth of a sibling who threatens to absorb the mother's attention is found with conspicuous frequency at the beginning of the asthmatic condition. For adults, sexual temptation or impending marriage may be a precipitating factor. For the young girl, the acceptance of the biological function of womanhood is the turning point in individual development, separating the girl from her mother. She becomes her mother's competitor instead of the dependent child. For the son the incestuous wishes threaten the dependent relationship to the mother. It has been found that most mothers of asthmatics are very sensitive to the manifestations of the son's physical attractions and react to them with withdrawal or even rejection. A combination of unconscious maternal seduction and overt rejection is one of the common findings in the history of asthma cases. Impending marriage in the adult son brings this conflict between the dependent attachment to the mother and the more mature sexual love for the fiancée to the fore and often marks the beginning of the asthmatic condition.

Hostile impulses directed against the love object may also

threaten the dependent relationship and provoke an attack. It appears also that any sudden effort which calls upon a person's independent functioning may revive the deep-seated conflict between independent and dependent tendencies and thus precipitate an attack.

In accord with these findings, the history of maternal rejection in the lives of asthma patients is found as a recurrent motif. The child who is still in need of maternal care naturally responds to maternal rejection with increased feelings of insecurity and increased clinging to the mother. In other cases, mothers of asthmatic children have been found to be insistent upon making their children prematurely independent. By pushing the child toward an as yet unacceptable independence, they achieve just the opposite; the result is an increased insecurity in the child and dependent clinging.

A condensed history of a twenty-two-year-old veteran suffering from asthma may concretely illustrate these psychodynamic formulations.

The first asthma attack developed when he returned for a furlough from the Pacific theater, where he served as an aviator. He had left for the Pacific front shortly after he was married and received his furlough after about eight months. On his arrival home he was met by his parents and his wife, and after a short stop at home with his parents he drove with his wife to a home which they received as a surprise present from the patient's father. The same night he awakened with a severe asthma attack, and he also had attacks during following nights. Laboratory studies found him allergic to a great many pollens, cat's hair, and house dust, but all attempts at desensitization failed completely. In the hospital he reacted favorably to a few psychiatric interviews with a woman social worker, and his attacks ceased for a short period. Then, when he heard that his mother was to undergo an operation, he had a relapse. After further psychiatric interviews during which he discharged violent emotion he improved again. By this time he was already released from the Army. He could not find work and so marked time by helping his father in his business. With the improvement in his asthmatic attacks, he became able to perform his duties in his father's business. When I interviewed him, he was working and supporting his family adequately. Only occasional mild attacks occurred at night. He gave me a vivid description of the events leading up to his first attack.

Returning from abroad, he was met at the station by his parents and wife and learned of the death of his next older brother, who was also in the Air Force. He was very fond of this brother, yet he did not react to the news of his death with any great emotion. He tried to account for this by the fact that for a while his brother was missing under circumstances which did not allow one to expect anything but the worst. He felt so confused when he met his family and was suddenly confronted with the fact of his brother's death that he almost forgot his wife was present. From the station they went for a short visit to the patient's home. The parents then suggested that he and his wife visit some friends. His wife drove the car, and instead of going to the friends, she drove to the new home, saying that the friends had moved. They arrived at the home, and in answer to their knock his father and mother came out from the house and handed the patient the key to their new home and immediately left, leaving him alone with his wife. He had mixed feelings about the whole situation and at first hesitated to accept this generous gift. He felt he had now taken his brother's place, as his father had always preferred the brother in the past. But then he decided to stay, and soon thereafter he and his wife had sexual intercourse. Then he fell asleep and later awoke with violent wheezing. Not knowing what had happened, he became terrified and thought he was about to die. The following night an even more severe attack occurred. He received treatment in a hospital, but this was completely ineffective. A careful anamnestic study revealed the following history.

The patient was a middle child of a middle-class family. His father was a lawyer of French ancestry. He had two brothers, four and six years older, and a sister five years younger. The brother next to him was strong and athletic; the patient was weak and scrawny. The brother was always preferred by the father; the mother wanted the patient to be a girl. When the sister was born, he felt he had lost the cherished position of the baby in the family. In spite of his physical handicaps, he played on the football team, did well in all athletics, and was very ambitious in his studies, and always ranked at the top of his class. At the beginning of the war his brother went into the Air Corps, and the patient soon followed him. Four days after he married he left for the front, where he participated actively in combat. At his own request he became a turret gunner after two of his friends were killed in the same capacity. He felt intense anxiety in combat but stuck it out "on account of his brother." On two occasions his plane was hit and he had a narrow escape. After a year of combat he came home for a furlough and his asthma attacks began as described.

In the patient's history, the central theme was his relationship to his brother, whom he both admired and envied. He remembered his father's preference for his brother. In his marital relationship, he was extremely demanding toward his wife. He wanted her to run the household efficiently as his mother did, and insisted upon the utmost cleanliness and order. He said he would have "checked out" immediately if his wife had not lived up to his standards.

At the time of my interview with him, he had a son, one and one-half years old, and his wife was again pregnant. He loved his son, who was sturdy, big-boned, and tough just like his brother, whose name he had given to the child. He reported two dreams to me. One had occurred the night before the interview; the other stuck in his mind vividly, although he had dreamed it about sixteen months before, the night after the birth of his son. In the more recent dream he saw his son jumping up from the breakfast table, grabbing the chandelier, and boldly swinging on it. The patient began to spank his son and awoke, hitting his wife. He said he would do the same in reality and added that his son was a tough little man, just like his brother. In the other dream he opened the trunk of his car, grabbed an instrument, and hurled it with all his strength as far as he could. This instrument had in reality annoyed him in the last few days by its rolling around at every turn of the car.

The actual meaning of this dream in the light of our extensive studies on asthma patients appears typical for asthmatics. It clearly expresses sibling rivalry, by the symbolic representation of the desire to eliminate the fetus from the maternal body (throwing the instrument out of the car). The patient obviously transferred to his son much of the feeling he had toward his sister, who had replaced him in the baby's position. The patient was dependent upon his wife, as we know. He reacted to his son with some unconscious jealousy, which he expressed in the dream in which he spanked his son. He also transferred to his son some of his attitudes toward his brother. Both were sturdy, aggressive, and foolhardy. Jumping and hanging from the chandelier was obviously an act of bravado about which he felt envious.

In the therapeutic interviews with the social worker, the patient immediately developed a strong dependent attachment and placed himself entirely in her hands. In these interviews he was able to express his feelings toward his brother and became aware of his competition with him; and for the first time in his life he openly expressed hostile feelings toward his father. Though he received great emotional relief from these interviews, they did not penetrate beyond his relation to his father and his brother; his feelings toward his mother and his wife were not uncovered. He was advised to continue treatment. From the history taken by the social worker and from my interview with the patient, the following psychodynamic factors can be reconstructed. The patient had a very strong dependent attitude toward the mother which he transferred to his wife. As a compensating defense against his dependent strivings, he developed a feeling of intense competition with his brother. This explains his extreme ambition in school and his behavior in the Army, which served as an overcompensation and denial of his passive dependent strivings and also served the purpose of winning parental love by outdoing his brother. His resentment against his sister was revived when his own son threatened his dependent position in relation to his wife. The psychological events after he returned home are quite transparent in the light of this emotional constellation. When he met his parents and wife at the station he completely overlooked the latter. Hearing about his brother's death meant for him unconsciously that he now became the object of parental love, and this provoked an unconscious feeling of guilt. His strongest desire after he returned home from the strains and deprivations of military service was to become the dependent child once again. A few hours later, he found himself alone with his wife in the new home. Everything was now emotionally reversed. The key to his new home symbolized the fact that he was on his own, separated from his parents, a mature man. He retreated emotionally from his task, and the longing to run back to mother was activated. The defense against this longing was the central factor precipitating the attack of asthma.

We are now ready to answer the question of why and how such a repressed desire for the mother should produce a spasm of the bronchioles, which is the physiological basis of the asthma attacks. On the basis of a psychoanalytic case study, the theory was advanced by E. Weiss (243) that the asthma attack represents a suppressed cry for the mother. Later Halliday also called attention to the relation of asthma to crying (109). This view has been further substantiated by the fact that most asthma patients spontaneously report that it is difficult for them to cry. Moreover, attacks of asthma have been repeatedly observed to terminate when the patient could give vent to his feeling by crying.

A further important observation is the immediate improvement occurring in a number of cases after the patient has confessed something for which he felt guilty and expected rejection (French and Johnson—90). Confession establishes the dependent attachment to the therapist which was disturbed by the patient's guilt feelings and expectations of being rejected. Speaking (confessing) is a more articulate use of the expiratory act by which the adult achieves the same result as the child does by crying. He regains the love of a person upon whom he depends. That suppression of crying leads to respiratory difficulties can be observed in the case of the child who tries to control his urge to cry or tries, after a prolonged period of futile attempts, to stop crying. The characteristic dyspnea and wheezing which appears strongly resembles an attack of asthma.

The recognition of emotional factors in asthma should not make one oblivious to the equally well-established influence of allergic factors. The latter are most conspicuous in seasonal attacks which appear simultaneously with the pollen to which the patient is sensitive. In cases where there is sensitivity to animal hair, paint, kapok, etc., attacks will often be produced with dramatic suddenness when the patient is exposed to the specific allergen in question. Desensitization is often effective in such cases.

The central problem is the relationship between the two kinds of etiological factor, between the emotional and the allergic.

First one must bear in mind that the asthmatic attack is a symptom, the immediate cause of which is a spasm of the bronchioles. On the basis of clinical evidence, there is no doubt that such a local spasm can be precipitated both by exposure to a specific allergen and by emotional factors of the nature described. It is most important to note that either factor alone may produce an attack but often both factors coexist. A great number of cases in the series of asthmatic patients studied in the Chicago Institute for Psychoanalysis showed some form of allergic sensitivity. Some of the patients retained this sensitivity after treatment as shown by skin tests, but lost their asthma. In such cases we are probably dealing with the phenomenon referred to in physiology as the "summation of stimuli"; in other words, only a combination of the emotional stimuli and the allergic factors will produce an attack. Separately the effect of either type of stimulus remains under the threshold of sensitivity of the "shock tissue"—in this case the wall of the bronchioles. This explains the not infrequent observation that after successful psychoanalysis, patients whose asthma attacks were restricted to the pollen season became, without any desensitization, resistant to their specific allergen. This theory also explains the claims of both psychiatrists and allergists regarding the therapeutic efficiency of their respective techniques. In most cases it is sufficient to remove one of the two coexisting causative factors, either the allergic or the emotional, in order to free the patient from his attacks. The untreated factor alone apparently does not suffice to produce an attack.

Whether or not the allergic and emotional factors should be considered independent of each other in their origin is still an open question. There are some indications that allergic predisposition and vulnerability in respect to the above-described conflict situation are related to each other in some unknown fashion. In other words, it is possible that the sensitivity to the "separation" trauma and to allergens frequently appear together in the same person and are parallel manifestations of the same basic constitutional factor.

Chapter XI

Emotional Factors in Cardiovascular Disturbances

1. DISTURBANCES OF HEART ACTION
(TACHYCARDIA AND ARRHYTHMIA)

THE SYMPTOMATOLOGY of the so-called functional cardiovascular disturbances in which emotional factors may be of etiological importance is manifold, such as tachycardia, nervous palpitation, different forms of arrhythmia and neurocirculatory asthenia, etc. No systematic clinical studies based on a precise psychodynamic investigation of both the emotional state and the somatic responses have been made. The close correlation of anxiety and rage with heart action is well known. Why these emotions, if they are permanently sustained as in the case of different psychoneuroses, particularly in anxiety states, manifest themselves in certain cases in tachycardia and in others in arrhythmia or symptoms of neurocirculatory asthenia is not established. It is probable that certain organic factors in the complex innervation of heart action by intrinsic ganglia and by central control are of great importance. The rigid distinction between organic and nervous (functional) disturbances of the heart is obviously a gross oversimplification. Certain organic factors which in themselves may be harmless may in combination with emotional disturbances produce symptoms of this kind. It is not infrequently found that patients in whom neurotic heart symptoms of long standing were diagnosed suddenly develop severe coronary disease. The interaction of organic and emotional factors is in some cases most intricate. Continued functional disturbance may favor development of organic lesions and slight organic defects and may perhaps favor the development of neurotic symptoms. So far as the specificity of the emotional factors is concerned, we can say only that chronic free-floating anxiety and repressed hostile impulses are the important emotion factors in such disturbances. Hostility stimulates anxiety, which, in the typical manner of neurotic vicious circles, increases the hostility. Such a neurotic nucleus may be present in a great variety of personalities but is perhaps more common in intimidated, inhibited personalities. Occasionally they can be observed in individuals suffering from a circumscribed type of phobic anxiety who otherwise appear quite active and aggressive. To select a certain psychological profile characteristic for patients suffering from functional heart symptoms is, we repeat, a futile undertaking.

2. ESSENTIAL HYPERTENSION

Essential hypertension is a clinical syndrome characterized by a chronic elevation of the blood pressure in the absence of a discernible organic cause. This syndrome has a progressive course from an early phase in which the blood pressure shows great lability and fluctuates markedly, to a later stage in which the blood pressure becomes stabilized at a high level, with, frequently, associated vascular and renal damage (Alexander, Fahrenkamp—7, 81).

The elevated arterial pressure in essential hypertension is attributed by most investigators to a widespread constriction of the arterioles throughout the vascular system. All efforts to discover a morphological basis for the vasoconstriction have failed. Although it is probable that chronic hypertension will in some instances produce vascular damage, the possibility also remains that such damage may be a concomitant rather than the result of the hypertension (Bradley—35).

Whether or not vascular damage ensues as a result of persistent hypertension, there is little to support the concept that the genesis of hypertension is associated with vascular lesions. The fact that the systemic circulation time remains normal (Weiss, Ellis—245), as does the blood flow (Abramson—5), favors the concept that a generalized increase in vasomotor tonus rather than some organic vascular change is responsible for the increased arterial pressure. Moreover, in the early phase of hypertension, left ventricle hypertrophy and lesions in the large vessels and arterioles are rarely found. In accord with this is the fact that patients with hypertension respond to a variety of life situations and physical stimuli with a further elevation of the blood pressure, as may be exemplified by the pressor responses of such patients to immersion of one hand in ice water (Page—177), to physical work (Barath—22), and to various other stimuli. Also, during the early phases patients frequently respond to psychotherapy with a fall of the mean blood pressure.

The increased vascular tonus which is responsible for the permanent elevation of blood pressure is the result either of an increase in vasomotor impulses to the smooth muscle of the arterioles or of some circulating pressor substance. Goldblatt's (101) demonstration that ischemia of the kidney results in the release of a chemical agent, renin, which is responsible for the conversion of a blood globulin to the pressor substance lent support to the concept that pressor agents acting directly on the smooth muscle of the vessels may be responsible for human hypertension. This led to a renewal of the many earlier attempts to demonstrate lesions in the renal vessels which may induce ischemia of the kidney and thereby be responsible for essential hypertension in man. In some instances such renal lesions which might induce renal ischemia have been found, but in the vast majority of instances, adequate changes are not present·in the kidney to account for the hypertension (Smith, et al.—214).

Since the blood vessels of the kidney are very reactive and respond with marked vasoconstriction to emotional and physical stimuli (Smith—213), it may be postulated that renal ischemia and a subsequent hypertension may result from such stimuli. The etiological problem is, then, to establish the nature of those neurogenic factors which produce the assumed functional changes in the circulation of the kidney responsible for the release of pressor agents. It is probable that continued neurogenic stimulation of the renal vessels may lead in time to minimal changes in the arterioles, the sum effect of which may amount to that of Goldblatt's clamp on the renal artery.

This neurogenic view is favored by the observation that the blood pressure of many patients with hypertension decreases during the transient blockade of the autonomic ganglia produced by tetraethylammonium chloride (TEAC). In a comprehensive study of the effect of TEAC on the blood pressure of patients with hypertension and various associated conditions, Ferris and his colleagues (85) noted that those with glomerulonephritis and toxemia of pregnancy gave insignificant responses to the administration of TEAC. However, about one-half of 105 patients with essential hypertension of various degrees of severity responded to blockade of the autonomic ganglia with a restoration of the blood pressure to normal levels. A high incidence of partial responses to TEAC was noted in the remainder of this group of patients. Further studies revealed that whereas 60 per cent of patients with essential hypertension consistently exhibit some response to repeated tests with TEAC, about 40 per cent responded at some times and did not at others. These studies reveal that the elevated arterial pressure of the majority of patients with essential hypertension is due to a neurogenic factor and that in a minority of instances a combination of neurogenic and humoral factors may be responsible.

Since the patients studied by Ferris and his colleagues varied markedly with respect to the severity and duration of the disease, it may well be that those patients who gave variable or little response to autonomic blockade were subjects in whom morphologic damage consequent to the hypertension had already taken place in the kidneys. In accord are the observations that patients with early or transient hypertension tend to have a greater incidence of positive responses to the administration of TEAC than those with more chronic forms of the disease. Equally significant is the observation that the most striking variations in the blood-pressure-reducing effect of autonomic blockade occur in relation to variations in emotional tension.

There appears to be little question of the fact that neurogenic factors play an important role in the maintenance of hypertension and even in the genesis of the syndrome. With the progression of the disease, tissue changes tend to play a greater and greater role. These changes favor the production of pressor substances, so that in the patient with a well-advanced hypertension the humoral factor may later become the dominant one. In the genesis of hypertension, however, precise knowledge of the neurogenic factors is the most important problem.

The literature is replete with numerous studies relating psychogenic factors with exacerbations of the hypertensive syndrome (Goldscheider; Mueller; Mohr; Fahrenkamp; S. Weiss; Fishberg; Schulze and Schwab; Moschcowitz; Riseman and S. Weiss—102, 172, 166, 81, 244, 87, 208, 169, 189). Many psychiatric studies demonstrate the influence of life situations on this syndrome (Alkan; Wolfe; K. Menninger; Dunbar;

Hill; Binger, *et al.;* E. Weiss—17, 256, 152, 73, 118, 32, 241). The majority of psychiatric studies emphasize the fact that inhibited hostile tendencies play an important role in this phenomenon, a fact which is in accord with Cannon's observation that fear and rage produce an increase in the blood pressure of the experimental animal. Cannon (43) demonstrated that with fear or rage there is an activation of the sympathetic nervous system and a secretion of epinephrine by the adrenal medulla, which in turn plays an important role in producing such physiological changes in the cardiovascular and other systems as may permit the organism to combat an attacker or to flee from the danger.

Systematic psychoanalytic studies have been performed on patients with hypertension. One such study revealed that chronic inhibited aggressive impulses which are always associated with anxiety markedly influence the blood-pressure level (Alexander—11). In spite of the fact that the group of patients consisted of individuals with many different types of personality, a common characteristic was their inability to express their aggressive impulses freely. Occasionally such patients would have outbursts of rage, but on the whole they maintained a remarkable degree of control, so that on superficial examination they gave the impression of well-adjusted, mature personalities. Indeed, quite frequently these patients were extremely compliant and agreeable and would go out of their way to please their associates.

Similar observations were made by Binger and his colleagues (32), who described what they regarded as typical family constellations in patients with hypertension. However, the marked variability in the life histories of such patients makes it improbable that a typical family background is characteristic. More probable is the hypothesis that a variety of past experiences result in the common characteristic of a repression of hostile impulses.

Illustrative of the patients studied at the Chicago Institute for Psychoanalysis is the businessman who presented himself as a modest, inconspicuous, polite person who never forced his way to the foreground (Alexander—11). He was ambitious, yet his desires to outdo his rivals were confined to his fantasies. His apparently modest, compliant attitude was particularly pronounced in his relations with his employer, whom he could not contradict. Typical of his reactions was the occasion when, as frequently occurred, the employer invited him to play golf the following Saturday. As usual, the patient accepted the invitation even though he preferred to play tennis with his own family at his club. Subsequently, when he left the office he was self-accusatory with respect to his inability to refuse his employer's invitations; rage and self-depreciation were concomitant.

Patients with hypertension are often inhibited sexually, and when they indulge in some illicit relationship it is connected with a great deal of anxiety and guilt because to them unconventional sexual activity means a protest and rebellion. A pronounced conflict between passive dependent or feminine tendencies and compensatory aggressive hostile impulses is revealed in the analysis of such individuals. The more they give in to their dependent compliant tendencies, the greater becomes their reactive hostility to those to whom they submit (Saul, Alexander—202, 7).

This hostility creates fear and makes them retreat from competition toward a passive dependent attitude. This, in turn, stirs up more inferiority feelings and hostilities, and a persistent vicious circle ensues. Noteworthy is the fact that the patient with hypertension cannot indulge freely in passive dependent wishes because of the conflict which they stimulate. The opposing tendencies of aggression and submission stimulate and block each other at the same time with a sort of emotional paralysis as a result.

Psychodynamic observations favor a psychosomatic view concerning the etiology of the generalized vasoconstriction characteristic of hypertension. Fear and rage are transient in both animals and man, and are associated with temporary physiological changes whereby the body becomes prepared for the concentrated effort involved in fight or flight. An increase in the arterial tension is one of the components of this physiological preparation. With the cessation of the fear-inducing situation, a return to normal ensues. In modern society, the free expression of hostility is prohibited; the individual is often antagonized but does not have the opportunity to express his aggressions freely in physical combat. Our society requires that the individual should have complete control over all his hostile impulses. While everyone is subjected to this restriction, some people are more inhibited in their faculty to express aggressive and self-assertive tendencies than are others in that they cannot make use even of such legitimate outlets for their aggressive impulses as are available. Consequently they live in a chronically inhibited hostile state. It may be assumed that chronically inhibited rage induced by such restrictions may lead to a chronic elevation of blood pressure because the rage cannot be discharged either in physical aggression or in some more sublimated form of self-assertive behavior. Thus, the hostile feelings which are not expressed may become the source of a permanent stimulation of the vascular system, as if the inhibited organism were constantly in preparation for a fight which never takes place (Fig. IV).

It may well be that when the inhibitions dictated by society and the prevalent cultures first begin to establish themselves in the individual who is a potential hypertensive, he begins to have fluctuations in the level of his blood pressure. Under the repetitive influence of vasomotor stimulation, the vascular system may begin to develop organic changes which do not become demonstrable for some time but which are reflected in the production of pressor agents, just as occurs in the dog when the renal arteries are clamped. Unfortunately this assumption is difficult to substantiate because the patient seldom comes to the physician's attention before or during the earliest phases of hypertension.

The individual who has become excessively inhibited under the influence of his early experiences will find it much more difficult to handle his aggressive impulses efficiently in adult life. He will tend to repress all his self-assertive tendencies and be unable to find some legitimate outlet for the expression of these tendencies. The damming up of his hostile impulses will continue and will consequently increase in intensity. This will induce the development of stronger defensive measures in order to keep the pent-up aggressions in check. The over-compliant, over-polite, submissive attitudes found in patients with hypertension are precisely such defenses, but they do not prevent the accumulation of tension. Consequently, feelings of inferiority develop which, in turn, stimulate aggressive impulses; and the vicious circle is perpetuated. Because of the marked degree of their inhibitions, these patients are less effective in their occupational activities and for that reason tend to fail in competition with others, so that envy is stimulated and their hostile feelings toward more successful, less inhibited competitors is further intensified.

The anamnestic study of the patient with hypertension usually reveals that at some time during the course of his development a relatively sudden change of temperament has occurred. The typical history is that the patient was very aggressive during early life and then, within the space of a short period of time, he began to act as if he were intimidated and meek. In many instances this change occurred during puberty. Sometimes such patients report that the change from belligerency to meekness took place as a result of a conscious effort; that they had to control themselves in order not to lose their popularity or because they had suffered defeats as a result of the expression of their aggressive impulses.

In accord with the concept that psychodynamic factors are the etiological basis of hypertension are the observations of

Figure IV.

Schematic illustration of specificity in the etiology of hypertension

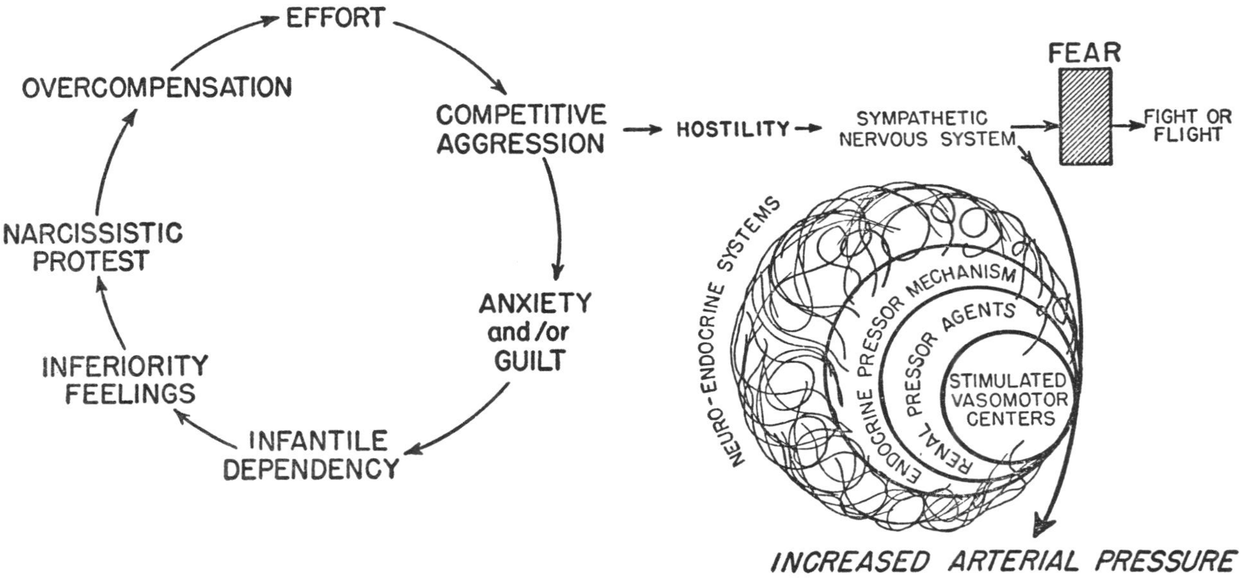

George Draper (67), who noted that with the development of certain neurotic symptoms, the blood pressure of some hypertensives fell to normal levels. Apparently the dammed-up hostile impulses could be released through the neurotic symptoms and they thus no longer served as the source of chronic excitation of vasomotor mechanisms.

Many writers have pointed out that hypertension is a disease of modern Western civilization. Schulze and Schwab (208), for example, found a statistically significant difference in the incidence of hypertension in African Negroes and Negroes in the United States. Whereas hypertension is extremely rare in African Negroes, the disease is common in the American Negro. Obviously a cultural factor rather than racial constitution must be responsible for this difference. It would appear that the difficulties inherent in the social adjustments which the American Negro must make induce the need for an extraordinary degree of self-control, which then becomes the crucial etiological factor.

The complete answer to the etiology of hypertension does not lie in elucidation of the psychodynamic factors only. Many neurotic persons reveal an inhibition of aggressive impulses and the typical conflict between passive dependent and aggressive competitive tendencies similar to the nuclear conflict of the patient with hypertension and yet do not develop an elevation of blood pressure. If the psychological factor alone were responsible for this disease one would expect to find that every patient who chronically inhibits his aggressive impulses and does not utilize some neurotic symptoms for the release of such impulses will develop hypertension. Actually this is not the case. As has been stressed repeatedly, only in combination with still unknown, possibly inherited somatic factors can psychodynamic influences produce chronic disturbances of the vegetative functions; and so it is in patients with hypertension. On the other hand, the possibility that hypertension is related to the inheritance of an unstable vasomotor system does not minimize the etiologic significance of psychodynamic factors.

Although several patients with hypertension have received psychoanalytic therapy, their number is still too small to permit statistical evaluation of the results. Nevertheless, it can be stated that the therapeutic results obtained with early hypertensive subjects are encouraging. Frequently the mean blood pressure of the patient becomes substantially reduced after psychoanalytic therapy has succeeded in making him more self-assertive; and such a patient may even become a problem to his environment. The relatives of such patients often remark that although the treatment may have improved the patient's physical status, it has made him a more difficult person to live with. As with many other conditions, prophylaxis is better than cure, and therefore it may be predicted that the most beneficial contribution to the problem of hypertension will come from earlier diagnosis and the application of psychotherapeutic measures to incipient cases.

Specific Dynamic Pattern in Essential Hypertension

Hostile competitive tendencies ——→ intimidation due to retaliation and failure ——→ increase of dependent longings ——→ inferiority feelings ——→ reactivation of hostile competitiveness ——→ anxiety and resultant inhibition of aggressive hostile impulses ——→ arterial hypertension.

3. VASODEPRESSOR SYNCOPE

Vasodepressor syncope, a disturbance of the cardiovascular system, has been subjected to careful psychosomatic study by Romano, Engel, et al. (191, 192, 78, 79, 80). The most common type of fainting, it may occur in healthy individuals when faced with an overwhelming danger, particularly in situations in which expression of fear has to be suppressed. It may occur with great frequency in certain neurotic individuals. The fainting is due to a sudden drop in blood pressure. The blood flow to the skin is decreased, and blood flow to the muscles is substantially increased. After an initial increase, the pulse rate becomes suddenly slow. Muscle tone and strength decrease and acute weakness follows.

There is good evidence to show that under the influence of danger, the physiological preparation for flight develops and the normal vasodilatation in muscles is a part of this adaptive response. On account of an inhibition of the flight reaction, the individual remains motionless and a kind of internal bleeding into the muscle system takes place, and a drop in blood pressure results. If this reaches the critical level, loss of consciousness occurs. It is important that the paralysis of motion occurs in erect position; in the recumbent position, fainting does not occur.

This condition can be readily differentiated from hysterical fainting in which fainting is a symbolic expression of psychological conflict. In hysterical fainting there are no changes in the cardiovascular system. Vasodepressor syncope is a typical example of a vegetative neurosis. The normal physiological response to fear is initiated, but on account of inhibition in voluntary behavior, the actual flight reaction is never consummated. The physiological response is interrupted after the initial period of preparation.

In its dynamics this phenomenon is analogous to other vegetative disturbances initiated by emotional factors. In peptic ulcer, the stomach prepares itself constantly for the intake of food. The initial phase of a physiological reaction takes place but the whole process is not consummated. The empty stomach is exposed continually to digestive secretions, which is one of the important pathogenic factors. In essential hypertension, on the other hand, the organism prepares itself for fight or flight with the normal physiological reaction. Action, however, is inhibited and therefore a homeostatic equilibrium is not regained as would occur after the fight or flight reaction had been fully carried out. In vasodepressor syncope, one specific phase of the flight reaction, the preparation of the muscle system for action by increased blood flow, is stimulated and then interrupted.

4. PSYCHOGENIC HEADACHES AND MIGRAINE

HEADACHES

Because of the extreme variety of etiological factors producing headaches it is commonly recognized in contemporary medical literature that headache is par excellence a symptom and not a disease entity. Disturbances in almost any organ system may precipitate, through reflex mechanisms, secondary physiological changes in the cranium which produce the subjective sensation of pain. Well-established causal factors are gastrointestinal disturbances—acute indigestion and constipation are leading in frequency—renal disease, hypertension, eyestrain, infection of the paranasal sinuses, liver and gallbladder disturbances, brain tumors. In all these cases headache is one of the sequelae of the basic condition.

The so-called histamine headache of allergic origin represents a rather distinct group. It can be reproduced experimentally by the injection of histamine.

The immediate pain-causing mechanisms vary, but changes in the caliber of the cranial blood vessels and alterations in the fluid content of the cranial cavity producing changes in intracranial pressure are recognized by most investigators as the principal factors. Locally the pain originates in the sympathetic fibers of the blood vessels; the brain substance proper is insensitive.

Apart from these reflex phenomena, the emotional origin of some headaches is well established. The literature abounds with reports that fatigue and emotional stress of all kinds may bring about headaches, which may assume the form of dull pain, pressure, pulsation, or other subjective sensations.

There are also reports, mostly by psychoanalysts, of single cases in which the headache is primary and appears as a conversion symptom with definite symbolic significance. As early as 1911, Sadger (201) reported recurrent headaches in a woman patient whom she treated psychoanalytically. The patient had three types of headache: pressure felt from outside, piercing headache, and pressure felt from within. The first type Sadger traced to an experience in infancy, being taken into bed by the father and feeling the tremendous weight and pressure of the father's body. The piercing headache originated from painful but also pleasurable masturbatory experiences with a girl friend when she was three or four years old; and the pressure headaches from within were based on early painful yet erotic experiences during defecation.

A male patient of Abraham's (2) expressed in his headaches feminine identification with his mother, who suffered from similar headaches. The headache gave the patient a passive masochistic gratification. Fenichel (83) described a case in which the headache symbolized threadworms which the patient had had as a child. The threadworms were connected in the unconscious with feces. The basis of the conversion symptom was the symbolic equation, feces = thoughts. In a case described by Seidenberg (209), a pulsating headache was the expression of repressed sexual desires symbolically representing erection. Gutheil (108) reports a patient whose migraine attacks terminated after sexual orgasm. Sometimes the patient would have several orgasms before relaxation and then the attack would end. I had the opportunity to study the headache of a middle-aged virgin, who felt the pain as an internal pressure threatening to burst her skull; this sensation was a symbolic expression of her repressed desire for pregnancy.

As conversion symptoms, headaches may obviously have a great variety of symbolic significances which are determined by the subjective needs of each individual patient. It is an open question whether in these conversion cases any underlying local physiological changes are present. They may belong to the category of sensory disturbances of a hysterical nature (psychogenic pain), in which are included paresthesias, hyperesthesias and anesthesias, in which no local changes are present and the whole process takes place in the higher sensory centers of the brain, manifesting itself merely in subjective sensations.

MIGRAINE

Migraine attacks constitute a well-defined group among the great variety of headaches. Whether or not their etiology is the same in every case, they represent a definite clinical entity as far as symptomatology and underlying physiological mechanisms are concerned. This makes possible comparative psychosomatic studies on migraine patients, a task almost insuperable with the heterogeneous group of patients suffering from other forms of headache.

The typical clinical manifestations of migraine attacks, such as their periodic nature, the prodromal disturbances (scotomata, occasional paresthesias, and speech difficulties), the fact that the pain is always unilateral, the presence of photophobia, vomiting, and nausea make the diagnosis clear-cut. Another characteristic feature is that after the attack the patient for a while enjoys a marked sensation of well-being. All these consistent features greatly facilitate comparative clinical studies on these patients. Still another fact which makes this disease entity suitable for psychosomatic studies is that the attacks often develop quite precipitously and sometimes terminate equally abruptly. This allows for the precise study both of the precipitating factors and of the factors responsible for the termination of the attack.

Physiological mechanisms

Vascular stretching is generally assumed to be one of the causes of pain in migraine. This is well substantiated by experimental studies of Graham and H. G. Wolff and co-workers (104, 47), who have shown that distension of the cranial arteries is responsible for the sensation of pain. This explains the highly specific beneficial effect of ergotamine tartrate, which produces vasoconstriction. It is commonly assumed that in histamine headaches of allergic origin the pain mechanism is the same. While the two mechanisms are similar, there are also distinct differences between the two types of headaches. The nature and the distribution of the pain are different; histamine headache is felt as a deeper pain, and it is always bilateral. Also the effect of ergotamine tartrate is much more pronounced in migraine attacks. Wolff explains this from the fact that histamine affects the intracerebral arteries, whereas ergotamine tartrate affects principally the branches of the external carotid, which are the ones involved in migraine.

The prodromal symptoms, the visual disturbances and paresthesias, are attributed to initial vasoconstriction, which induces the attack. Wolff considers the vasodilatation as an overcompensatory reaction against the initial vasoconstriction. In my opinion the vasodilatation may have an independent origin, which will be discussed later (page 162).

Emotional factors

The outstanding etiological significance of emotional factors in migraine has been recognized by a great number of authors. These observations pertain partly to typical precipitating factors and partly to personality traits common to patients inclined to have migraine headaches. Touraine and Draper (235) described a "constitutional" personality type characteristic of the migrainous individual. Physically these patients show acromegaloid traits; in personality make-up they have a retarded emotional development but superior intelligence. Their sexual adjustment is unsatisfactory. According to these authors, migraine headaches first appear when the patients lose the protection of home and have to face the responsibilities of living alone. They note an exaggerated dependence upon the mother, from whom they can never emancipate themselves.

Olga Knopf (133) studied thirty patients, twenty-two of whom were women. She described them as belonging to the "goody-goody" type; they were ambitious, reserved, relaxed, dignified, sensitive, domineering, and devoid of a sense of humor. The women all had poor heterosexual adjustment.

None of the authors mentioned go further in their descriptions than the enumeration of certain isolated personality features. They do not attempt to discern any underlying psychodynamic patterns.

Of greater importance are the thorough studies of Fromm-Reichmann (96), who treated eight migraine patients with intensive psychotherapy. She found that in these patients hostile, envious impulses originally directed against intellectually brilliant persons were turned against the self through the well-known guilt mechanisms.

Harold Wolff (257), in addition to his fundamental work on the physiology of migraine attacks, has made careful studies of typical personality features of such patients. He stressed compulsive characteristics, perfectionism, ambition, excessive competitiveness, rigidity, and inability to delegate responsibility. According to Wolff, these patients have a chronic resentful attitude which results from their inability to keep up with compulsively assumed responsibilities to live up to their perfectionistic ambitions. This frustrated attitude results in tension and fatigue until some external event further aggravates their ever-present resentfulness and precipitates a migraine headache. H. Selinsky (210) came to similar conclusions. He too stressed the significance of "struggle, resentment and anxiety." The attack occurs when the patient faces a task beyond his ability.

There is considerable clinical evidence that a great number

of patients suffering from migraine headaches show these surface attitudes characteristic for the so-called compulsive character types. More impressive, however, is the uniformity of the precipitating emotional factors.

Most of the publications on the psychology of migraine headaches, both earlier and more recent, mention the presence of repressed or suppressed hostile impulses. (Weber; Brenner, Friedman and Carter; Rosenbaum; Fromm-Reichmann; Wolff; Eisenbud; Wolberg; Johnson—239, 36, 194, 96, 257, 77, 255, 125.) Psychoanalysts who treat migraine patients in frequent interviews have repeated opportunity to observe the beginning or the termination of a migraine attack during the session. The common introduction of the migraine attack is a state of repressed rage. The most striking observation is the sudden termination of the attack almost from one minute to another after the patient becomes conscious of his hitherto repressed rage and gives expression to it in abusive words.

Such observations leave little doubt that repressed hostile impulses have a direct and specific correlation with migraine attacks. The relevance of the characteristic personality features reported by the various authors consists merely in that personality types that are likely to repress their hostile impulses have a greater inclination toward migraine attacks. This explains such findings as that the inhibited person, the reserved "goody-goody" type described by Knopf or the compulsive personality noted by Wolff, are commonly found among sufferers from migraine. Repressed hostility, however, is an extremely common feature among many kinds of persons. This confronts us once again with the crucial question of specificity in psychosomatic research. What are the specific psychodynamic factors responsible for the fact that one inhibited patient develops hypertension, another arthritis, and a third migraine headache?

It is possible that in migraine headaches the same condition obtains which was noted in hypertension—namely, the absence of specific psychoneurotic symptoms suitable for draining off pent-up hostile impulses. Even if this turns out to be correct, the question of choice of somatic symptom still remains unanswered. Fromm-Reichmann's observation that the hostile, envious attitude in these cases is specifically directed against intellectual achievement may be of significance concerning the choice of organ. The familial nature of migraine headaches, which has been recognized by most clinicians, points to constitutional factors which probably pertain to individual peculiarities of cerebral circulation.

The coincidence of migraine and hypertension on the one hand and migraine and epilepsy on the other is also of importance in this connection. Headache is sometimes a secondary symptom of hypertension. This coincidence, however, may have both a constitutional and a psychodynamic basis. In all three diseases—epilepsy, hypertension, and migraine—destructive, hostile impulses play an important role. Freud's view of the epileptic attack as a short-circuited, unco-ordinated discharge of destructive impulses is substantiated by certain fugue states which appear as epileptic equivalents and in which the patients become destructive, often homicidal in their behavior. Migraine attacks may also appear occasionally as epileptic equivalents.

In respect to specificity of the precipitating psychodynamic factors, the nature of the hostile impulses is important. A fully consummated aggressive attack has three phases. At first there is the preparation of the attack in fantasy: its planning and its mental visualization. This is the *conceptual phase.* Second, there is the vegetative preparation of the body for concentrated activity: changes in metabolism and blood distribution. Blood flows in greater quantity to the organs needed in concentrated attack—skeletal muscles, lungs, and brain. This is the *phase of vegetative preparation.* Finally there is the *neuro-muscular phase,* the consummation of the aggressive act itself through muscular activity.

Possibly the nature of the physical symptoms depends upon the phase which is accentuated or in which the whole psycho-physiological process of hostile aggression becomes arrested. If the inhibition takes place as early as the psychological prep-aration for an aggressive attack, a migraine attack develops. If the second phase, the vegetative preparation for the attack, develops but the process does not progress further, hyperten-sion follows. And finally if the voluntary act is inhibited only in the third phase, an inclination toward arthritic symptoms or vasomotor syncope may develop. Further precise psycho-dynamic studies are needed to test the validity of this hy-pothesis, which is strongly favored by the observation that migrainous persons are primarily "thinkers" and not "doers," while arthritics have a strong inclination toward muscular activity.

According to Cannon, the blood flow to the brain remains ample and is relatively increased in states of violent emotion. In inhibited rage, when muscle action is blocked and blood flow to the muscles does not increase, while the splanchnic area empties, the blood flow to the cranium probably becomes even greater. This may be the physiological basis of the mi-graine attacks. Increased muscle tonus and elevation of blood pressure are other components of the rage syndrome. The above hypothesis tries to account for the fact that in the state of inhibited rage certain patients respond with one and others with another component of the total physiological syndrome of rage.

The therapeutic problem of migraine has two aspects—the management of the attacks themselves and the prevention of recurrence.

For checking the attack, there seems to be general agree-ment concerning the therapeutic effectiveness of ergotamine tartrate. Its beneficial effect is due to its vasoconstricting influence.

The larger problem of prevention is directed toward eliminating the causes of the local disturbance of the cranial circulation. Marcussen and Wolff (147) report good results with environmental management and advice to the patient. They study the particular circumstances which precipitate attacks and make the patients aware of these conditions, guide them in making the necessary changes in their mode of living, occupational, recreational, and interpersonal. In two-thirds of the cases they had more or less favorable results with this type of therapy.

The most penetrating therapeutic approach is provided by psychoanalysis, which attempts to achieve a resolution of fundamental conflicts and a change in the patient's ability to handle emotional tensions, particularly unconscious, hostile impulses. Fromm-Reichmann psychoanalyzed eight patients and obtained satisfactory results in the majority of cases. Johnson has described in detail the psychoanalytic treatment of a case with good results.

Chapter XII

Emotional Factors in Skin Diseases

SYSTEMATIC studies in the field of skin diseases are still lacking, although a great many more or less disconnected observations are reported in the literature. For a comprehensive review of the literature, the reader is referred to an article by Stokes and Beerman (221).

That the skin is an important organ for expressing emotion is well known. The best-known examples are blushing in shame, and itching as a sign of impatience. The skin, constituting the surface of the body, is the somatic locus of exhibitionism. Certain reflex changes in the skin, such as pallor, flushing, and perspiration, are constituent parts of the emotional states of rage and fear. The pylomotor response to anxiety is particularly prominent in cats, but is present also in human beings, as revealed by such expressions as "a hair-raising story."

The skin is also an important sensory organ and, as such, is affected by conversion symptoms—e.g., anesthesias, paresthesias, and hyperesthesias. And finally, in the psychology of the skin the sensation of pain has a central place. Masochistic tendencies must therefore have a close affinity to the skin. Ac-

cording to Joseph V. Klauder (132), "The psyche exerts a
greater influence on the skin than any other organ. . . . The
skin is an important organ of expression of emotions comparable only to the eye." He lists the following skin conditions
in which "psychologic phenomena either play a motivating
role or are a notable determining factor":

Blushing
Pallor
Cutis anserina } motivated by emotions
Horripilation
Changes in secretion of sweat
(Dermatographia—angioneurosis—erythematous eczema—an-
    gioneurotic edema—acute eczema (acute dermatitis)
Urticaria, acute or chronic
Edema (angioneurotic edema, edema in hysterics)
Pruritus, localized or generalized
Phobias referable to the skin
Neurotic excoriations: dermatothlasia (Fournier), self-produced
    lesions (no deception intended; variable psychogenesis)
Dermatitis factitia (mythomania of Dupre—self-produced lesions
    for deception)
Fixed pain and sensory disturbances (topalgias of Blocq, for ex-
    ample, "burning tongue")
Angiospasm (so-called "dead" fingers)
Sudden loss of hair (alopecia areata) or a sudden turning to
    white (canities)
Trichotillomania
Trichokryptomania
Stigmas of the crucifixion
Tattoo
Psychogenically produced manifestations in the allergic state.

The best-established clinical observations of skin manifestations as a part of neurotic symptomatology comprise such
conditions as neurodermatitis, eczema, angioneurotic edema,
urticaria, and pruritus. Some authors also mention emotional
factors in seborrhea, pompholyx and psoriasis. As early as
1916, Jelliffe and Evans (124) described a case of psoriasis
in which they asserted that psychological factors—i.e., ex-

hibitionistic trends—had a primary etiological significance. Attempts at generalizations are not yet successful. All that can be said is that in eczema and neurodermatitis, sado-masochistic and exhibitionistic trends have a rather specific correlation to the skin symptoms (Miller—157). I observed in several cases the following dynamic pattern. Showing the body in order to obtain attention, love, and favor—in other words, exhibitionism—is used as a weapon in competition, and arouses guilt feelings. According to the talion principle, the punishment should be commensurate with the crime; the skin which served as the tool of exhibitionism becomes the place of a painful affliction. F. Deutsch and R. Nadell (62) also observed narcissistic and exhibitionistic traits.

Scratching is of great etiological significance in these diseases. Psychoanalytic studies show that the important factor in scratching is the hostile impulse, which, on account of guilt feelings, is deflected from its original target and is turned against one's own self. (Miller, Bartemeier, Scarborough—158, 23, 205). Illustrative is the following case study by Spiegel in the Chicago Institute for Psychoanalysis.

The patient, a 22-year-old white, single girl, was referred for treatment because of recurrent bouts of severe neurodermatitis. The lesions, which occurred mostly on the face and upper and lower extremities, were eczematoid in type, consisting of discrete, red, raw, itching areas. The patient scratched the lesions furiously, especially during her sleep, until they wept and bled, so that she was often quite disfigured. She had seen a number of dermatologists and had frequently been told that she could not be helped because the condition was due to emotional factors, a conclusion she herself had drawn on the basis of wide psychological reading.

The skin lesions had been present on and off all of the patient's life. She had first developed eczema a week after her birth. Her mother had been very disturbed during the pregnancy by the accidental death of her seven-year-old son, and subsequently by desertion and divorce by her husband. The patient's childhood was spent in the homes of various relatives, where she always felt insecure because of her mother's timidity and her depreciated status of almost a servant in the household. The patient was shy and socially backward in school, but bright and alert in her studies. She suffered greatly from feeling "different" and unwanted because of the recurrent eczema and the lack of a father and a normal family life. In college, however, with physical maturity, she blossomed out and became popular socially. After graduation she found a good job, and began to form intense attachments to various men. The attachments were always broken off with the appearance of a severe attack of eczema. It was when this recurrent pattern threatened her job and normal interpersonal relations that her dawning insight brought her to treatment.

Psychoanalytic therapy was initiated, and she developed almost immediately an explosive masochistic transference neurosis. Simultaneously with an exacerbation of the skin lesions, the patient showed in every way that she expected to be rejected by the therapist, and that she felt guilty because of both hostile and erotic transference feelings. These feelings she displaced to a series of relations with men, characterized by an immediate gratification of sexual impulses, and followed by depression and guilt and hostility when she learned that the man had no intention of marrying her. It was always at this point that the skin lesions reached their height. In the course of the analysis it became clear that the patient turned to the therapist (or some other man) as the long-lost father. To these father substitutes she turned with a dependent oral craving and with the wish for warm, cozy, generalized musculocutaneous "cuddling." When frustrated in these wishes she reacted with hostility and guilt. This was handled partly by projection of the blame in the formula "all men are bastards," and partly by expression of the affects in the skin. She expressed her hostile feelings by scratching, and the resulting disfigurement represented shame, humiliation, and rejection. At this point, feeling completely unlovable, the patient would attempt to establish a closer relation with her mother, and when this failed, would enter a period of depression. The cycle was brought to a close by the appearance of a masculine protest, much attention to her job, a turning away from close ties to women and men, and a lightening of affect and clearing of the skin.

During the course of a three-year period of treatment, the

patient slowly developed insight into this repetitive pattern, and eventually was able to form a non-masochistic relation with a man whom she ultimately married. With the reduction of guilt and hostility, she was able to allow herself satisfaction in this relationship, and the skin lesions cleared and have not recurred.

In urticaria, a specific correlation to suppressed weeping has been described by Saul and Bernstein (203), and confirmed by the several cases which I had opportunity to study. As in asthma, to which urticaria has an intrinsic relationship, both clinically and psychodynamically, inhibited dependent longing for a parental object is a conspicuous finding. This, together with the fact that many urticaria patients cannot weep easily and that urticaria attacks are often suddenly terminated by a weeping spell, is further indication of an intimate relationship between suppressed weeping and urticaria. In one analyzed case of angioneurotic edema, Lorand (143) observed a strong early fixation to dependent desires combined with pronounced sibling rivalry. Kepecs, Robin, and Brunner (130) recently corroborated through experimental studies the correlation of fluid secretion in the skin with weeping. They raised a blister in the skin by cantharides and observed in it a sharp rise in the fluid level associated with weeping. Emotionally caused increase in fluid secretion in skin patients can be reduced by psychotherapy, abreaction, and antihistaminic drugs.

In different forms of pruritus, particularly pruritus ani and vulvae, and also in some other dermatoses, inhibited sexual excitement is an important psychodynamic factor. In these cases, scratching is a source of conscious erotic pleasure and is clearly a masturbatory equivalent (Stokes, Gillespie, Cormia and Slight—220, 100, 51).

In all itching skin conditions, a vicious circle takes place. Continued scratching leads to changes in the delicate structure of the skin, which makes the sensory endings more sensitive to external stimuli (lichenization). Thus, a somatic source is added to the psychological stimulus for scratching. This perpetuates scratching, which in turn increases the structural changes which cause itching.

Effective therapy of such skin conditions requires a coordinated psychological and somatic treatment. In many cases mechanical prevention of scratching by different protective measures, particularly during the night, is indispensable to break the cycle. Psychotherapy at the same time attacks the underlying emotional factors.

Chapter XIII

Emotional Factors in Metabolic and Endocrine Disturbances

1. THYROTOXICOSIS

THE PSYCHOLOGICAL factors in thyrotoxicosis (Basedow's or Graves' disease), as well as many of the physiological mechanisms involved, are well established. Hence this disease is especially appropriate for the study of psychosomatic interrelations.

Various manifestations of emotional tension may precede the development of the clinical syndrome. Thus, 28 per cent of Maranon's (145) 159 patients with hyperthyroidism volunteered the information that their disease was precipitated by some emotional upheaval, and Conrad (49) found evidence of psychic traumata in 94 per cent of 200 patients. Similar observations have been reported by many investigators (Bram; Goodall and Rogers; Moschcowitz; Wallace; Mittelmann—38, 103, 170, 238, 164). In fact, some of the earlier students of the problem were so impressed with the significance of psychic factors as precipitating agents as to postulate that some severe emotional shock may be responsible for the development of a form of hyperthyroidism which was designated as "Shock-Basedow." In this connection Moschcowitz noted the frequency with which an emotional crisis involving a large group of persons may precipitate the disease in many individuals.

Apart from their etiological significance, emotional changes constitute an important part of the symptomatology. In addition to thyroid enlargement, exophthalmos, sweating and tremor, tachycardia, elevated B.M.R. and blood iodine, diarrhea, and other signs of autonomic imbalance, there are characteristic psychological changes, such as irritability, mood swings, sleeplessness, and anxiety, which constitute integral parts of the total clinical picture. These emotional changes can be induced by the administration of excessive amounts of thyroid hormone and can therefore be considered the direct result of thyroid hyperfunction. Other symptoms—as will be discussed later—are neurogenic. The cause of the thyroid hyperfunction is not yet fully established, but its effects have been well known since Horsely succeeded in curing symptoms of myxedema by administration of thyroid extract. The effects obtained by this substitution therapy are equally dramatic in producing bodily as well as psychological changes. They demonstrate that normal mental functioning, particularly the speed of mental processes, is dependent upon normal thyroid secretion. The lethargic, retarded, and intellectually dull personality of the myxedema patient is in sharp contrast with the highly alert, oversensitive, anxious character of the hyperthyroid patient.

It appears, then, that the interrelationship between the psychological processes and thyroid functions is a reciprocal one. Thyroid secretion accelerates mental functions, increases alertness and sensitivity, and thus predisposes to anxiety; but at the same time emotional experiences have an effect upon thyroid secretion itself.

PHYSIOLOGY

The accelerating influence of thyroxin is not restricted to psychological processes; it is also the regulator of the rate of metabolism. The precise nature of the hormone of the thyroid gland is still doubtful, although it has been established that circulating inorganic iodine which is taken up by the gland is converted into an organically bound form and a considerable portion of it is secreted as a protein containing thyroxin (thyroglobulin). Thyroxin accelerates metabolism and circulation, which manifests itself in increased heart rate, increased heat production and oxidation, increased appetite, and loss of weight. The precise mechanism whereby this is accomplished is not yet established. The thyroid hormone has an important role in the process of growth. Phylogenetically it appears first in amphibians, where its normal function is the acceleration of metamorphosis. Artificial administration of thyroxin advances the salamander from an aquatic to a land existence, from gill to lung breathing. The phylogenetic progress from amphibian to land existence is due to the development of the thyroid gland.

In the higher vertebrates thyroxin is instrumental in the process of maturation, as demonstrated by the fact that absence of thyroxin in myxedema not only produces mental retardation but also delays the ossification of the epiphysis of the long bones. With good reason Brown (39) called it the "gland of creation." He called attention to the fact that "the position and arrangement of the uterus in Limulus (Horseshoe Crab) closely resembles that of the thyroid with its thyroglossal duct in Ammocetes (Larval Lamprey), one of the most primitive of the vertebrates." Gaskell (97, 98) referred to the same fact in finding "the relationship which has been shown from time immemorial to exist between the sexual organs and the thyroid in man and other animals and has hitherto been a mystery without any explanation, may possibly be the last reminiscence of the time when the thyroid glands were uterine glands of the paleostracan ancestor."

The fact that normally during pregnancy the thyroid gland is enlarged and increases its activity is further evidence indicating the role of the thyroid in the processes of both growth and procreation (Soule—217). This is supported by such observations as that of King and Herring (131) that hypothyroid patients are often sterile and have an increased tendency to abortion. In this connection it is also significant that according to Kenneth Richter (188) hyperthyroidism produces an increase in the discharge and transference of germinal products through efferent genital ducts. This indicates that also in the male the thyroid hormone has a positive influence upon procreative functions.

This large array of observations from the fields of clinical pathology, endocrine physiology, embryology, and genetics leads to the following conclusions: The product of the thyroid gland, thyroxin, is primarily a stimulator of cell metabolism, and as such it favors intellectual growth and performance, increases sensitivity, alertness, and, in its extreme form, anxiety, and also stimulates general growth and the procreative processes. Increased function requires increased metabolism; hence it can be assumed that increased bodily accomplishments require increased thyroid secretion. It appears, however, that the specific function of the thyroid consists in its prolonged stimulating effect when the body is called upon to perform long-term accomplishments, for example during pregnancy. Growth also is a long-term accomplishment of the organism. Thyroxin and the growth hormone of the anterior pituitary are synergists. This long-term effect of thyroxin is in contrast with the short-term effect of adrenin in emergency situations which require sudden concentrated effort. The injection of thyroxin has an effect over days, while the effect of adrenin injection lasts only a few minutes. Yet adrenin and thyroxin are synergists, and patients with thyrotoxicosis are more sensitive to adrenin (Crile—52).

The function of the thyroid, however, can be fully under-stood only in its complex interrelation with other endocrine glands. With the exception of those instances in which there is

an actively secreting tumor of the thyroid gland, the cause of
the pathological rate of thyroglobulin production appears to
lie outside the gland. The weight of evidence indicates that
the increased secretion of the thyroid is due to a thyroid-
stimulating (thyrotropic) hormone of the anterior pituitary
gland. The excessive production of thyrotropic hormone produces the hyperplasia of the thyroid gland and hypersecretion
of the thyroid hormone. Further, the thyrotropic hormone or
some closely related hormone is responsible also for the
exophthalmos observed in patients with Graves' disease, a
phenomenon which is independent of the presence of the
thyroid.

Ordinarily the rate of secretion of the thyrotropic hormone
of the anterior pituitary gland is controlled by the amount of
hormone produced by the thyroid itself. However, in thyrotoxicosis this control is absent, so that the thyrotropic hormone is secreted in excessive amounts without any check, as is
revealed by the high concentrations of this hormone in the
blood of some patients with exophthalmic goiter (De Roberts
—60). The removal of the thyroid gland or the administration of antithyroid drugs to the patient with hyperthyroidism
may reduce the production of thyroxin and most of the symptoms of hyperthyroidism, yet the thyrotropic hormone may
actually increase (Soffer, et al.—215) and the exophthalmos
may progress.

Little is known concerning the precise mechanism whereby
thyrotropic hormone production is accelerated in hyperthyroidism. It may well be that some mechanism similar to that
postulated by Selye and extended by Long and others is responsible for the excessive activity of the pituitary gland (Figure V). Accordingly, a variety of stresses, chemical, toxic,
nervous, and emotional, may activate the anterior pituitary
gland either through a direct effect on the hypothalamus or
secondarily through activation of the sympathico-medullo-
adrenal system. In accord are Soffer's observation that the ad-

ministration of epinephrine can result in an increased secretion of thyrotropic hormone (215) and Uotila's (236) observa-

FIGURE V.

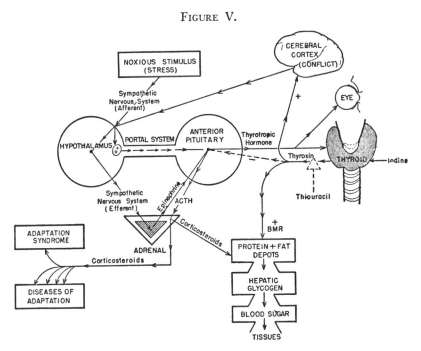

Mechanisms that may be involved in the production and maintenance of hyperthyroidism are illustrated schematically. Activation of the hypothalamus may result in (1) an increased secretion of epinephrine and a subsequent stimulation of the anterior pituitary by the increased circulating epinephrine, and/or (2) the secretion of some humoral agent by the hypothalamus which is then transported to the anterior pituitary. Stimulation of the anterior pituitary results in increased production of thyrotropic hormone with a subsequent stimulation of the thyroid gland. The reciprocal relation between the thyroid and anterior pituitary is illustrated. (Mirsky.)

tion that cutting the stalk of the rat will prevent the hypertrophy of the thyroid which follows upon exposure to cold.

All this indicates that thyrotoxicosis is not a local condition of the thyroid gland. Thyroid secretion is only an effector link in the chain of physiological processes; it is controlled by the thyrotropic hormone of the anterior pituitary gland, which itself is under sympathetic and eventually hypothalamic control. Through corticothalamic pathways psychological processes exert their influence upon hypothalamic control of the pituitary gland and as a last link upon thyroid activity.

We turn our attention now to the specific nature of the psychological stimuli upon thyroid activity.

PSYCHOSOMATIC OBSERVATIONS

Hyperthyroidism may be precipitated by a variety of factors, but the most common is psychic trauma or intense emotional conflict. The importance of emotional factors is borne out by the constancy with which emotional disturbances precede the onset of the illness and by the striking similarity of the emotional factors and the personality structure of the patients.

A number of investigators have reported upon the psychodynamics of the hyperthyroid patient. Lewis (138, 139) was impressed by the marked incestuous fixation upon the father which was exhibited by hyperthyroid women and by the prevalence of impregnation fantasies. The only man that Lewis studied revealed homosexual cravings and resembled the women because of a marked inverted oedipus complex based on a feminine identification.

The analysis of three women with hyperthyroidism impressed Conrad (49) with their extreme dependence upon the mother, their fear of losing affection and shelter and of the burdens that are involved in assuming the maternal role, and the resulting difficulty of making an identification with the mother. Conrad also studied a great number of patients anamnestically and found a statistically significant incidence of losing the mother during early infancy, especially during childbirth. Some of the male patients also revealed an excessive dependence upon their mothers. It would appear that the specific factor common to all the patients is their difficulty in exchanging the role of being nursed for that of nursing.

Lidz also observed unusual attachment to a parent in twelve of his patients (140).

Mittelman's findings in sixty patients were less specific. He emphasized an exaggerated dependence upon the parents and strict standards. He noted the role of trauma which affects the patient's psychologically sensitized spots.

Brown and Gildea (40) were impressed by the similarity of characteristic personality features which were present before the onset of the clinical syndrome in the fifteen patients that they studied. They noted that the patients had extreme feelings of personal insecurity, a strong sense of responsibility, and a tendency to control the outward expression of emotions, and that any threat to their security, either by prolonged strain or by sudden emotional shock, could precipitate the hyperfunction of the thyroid gland. Although these authors do not emphasize it, an impressive struggle against insecurity, with attempts to master it by one's own efforts, is apparent in the reported histories of their patients.

Anamnestic interviews of twenty-four patients conducted by Ham, Carmichael, and Alexander (116), together with members of a psychosomatic seminar in the Psychiatric Department of the University of Illinois and the psychoanalytic study of one patient at the Chicago Psychoanalytic Institute by Ham, confirm the findings of the previous investigators. Particularly is this so with reference to the significance of fear and anxiety, the marked dependence upon parental figures, and the excessive insecurity, and also the opposite trends of efforts toward assuming responsibility, achieving maturity, becoming self-sufficient, and taking care of others. The main objective of this study was to identify the characteristic psychodynamic pattern in which these various psychological factors are related to each other. Careful analysis of the data revealed a psychodynamic pattern which appears to be common in both men and women with hyperthyroidism. Threat to security in early childhood or infancy appeared to be the dynamic nucleus and was frequently related to pronounced fears of death, to which most of these patients had been exposed early in their lives. This is in accord with Conrad's demonstration of a high incidence of the loss of the mother during early life. However, that was not the only source of fear and insecurity; an unhappy marriage of the parents, instability of personality in one of the parents, parental rejection, extreme forms of economic stress, birth of a younger sibling in large families which led to actual neglect, and still other life situations served as sources of the fear and insecurity which the patients exhibited.

Threat to security in childhood is a very common finding both in neurotics and in healthy individuals. Characteristic of patients with thyrotoxicosis is their manner of handling this insecurity. Because of the external circumstances described above, these patients cannot overcome their anxiety by turning to their parents for help. Their dependent needs are constantly frustrated by fate or by parental attitudes, by loss of one or both parents, or by parental rejection, as well as by conflicts of more complex nature which involve guilt. Since they are frustrated in their dependent needs, they make a desperate attempt to identify themselves prematurely with one of the parents, usually the mother. ("If I cannot have her, I must become like her, so that I can dispense with her.") This precocious identification is beyond their physiological and psychological capacity and results in a persistent struggle to master the anxiety and insecurity by a pseudo self-reliance. This trait was observed by Conrad, who described it as an inability to live up to maternal standards which these patients vainly seek to reach. Brown and Gildea observed the same phenomenon when they noted the paradoxical coexistence of insecurity and effort to assume responsibility. Also Ruesch, et al. (200), noted the fact that these patients were frequently forced by life circumstances to take premature responsibilities.

The constant struggle against anxiety may be manifested by denial, a kind of counterphobic attitude: a compulsive urge to undertake those activities which are most feared. This may account for the urge to seek responsibility and to be helpful, in spite of underlying insecurity and dependence. In a number of patients the most outstanding character trait, present from childhood, was the assumption of the dutiful role of motherhood in that they became second mothers for the other siblings.

The same emotional contradiction appears in different forms—the compulsive urge to become pregnant in spite of the fear of pregnancy, or the attempt to master fear by self-sufficiency, which the patient tries to achieve by identification with the person toward whom the frustrated dependent desires are directed. Likewise, fear of death is mastered by a wish to give life to children. The loss of the mother is combatted by becoming a mother. This may express itself in pregnancy fantasies, as was noted by Nolan Lewis. It is this constant effort to master anxiety which accounts for the high incidence of phobias in the history of hyperthyroid patients (Ficarra and Nelson—86).

A unique and striking feature is the frequency of dreams of death, caskets, ghosts, and dead persons which these patients report spontaneously.

A strong repression of hostile impulses resulting from extreme dependence was observed in the Chicago study and also by Ruesch, *et al.* The assumption of a motherly, protective attitude toward younger siblings frequently represents an overcompensation for sibling rivalry and requires the repression of hostility. Protecting the younger siblings gives a vicarious gratification for the patient's own dependent needs and also expiates guilt derived from rivalry.

The pseudo maturity, the exaggerated effort to assume the

maternal role through frequent pregnancies and excessive care of others, the counterphobic attitudes—all reflect the attempt of the patient with hyperthyroidism to master anxiety by self-sufficiency. This constant effort toward self-sufficiency, the patient's need to become prematurely independent, can be explained by the fact that the anxiety induced by a threat to security in early childhood could not be alleviated by dependence upon others.

These features are illustrated by the following excerpts from case histories: [1]

A striking example of early insecurity caused by the death of parents and exposure to other death episodes is shown in the case of D.B., a 32-year-old white widow who, in addition to experiencing extreme poverty as a child, had been treated harshly by her stepfather following the divorce of her parents. When she was four, she saw a woman burned to death. At eight years of age she saw a coffin tipped over by accident and the corpse of a little friend, a three-year-old girl, fell out on the floor. She witnessed the suicide of her grandfather as well as the death of her grandmother. The horror of these events is still vivid in her mind. Later in life her husband died, forcing her to support the family.

Examples of premature need for self-sufficiency, manifested in active participation in the support of the family or in taking care of younger siblings, follow:

B.R., a 13-year-old white girl, is described by the mother as a "little old lady" because she is so prematurely grown-up, obedient, and reliable. She learned to cook when she was six and has cooked and helped with the housework ever since. Whenever her mother became ill she swept and cleaned the house and took care of the whole family. She acted as second mother to her younger brother.

H.D., a 35-year-old-single man, the last of eight children, is the only surviving male. Two older brothers died at age 10 and 3 respectively, and one brother died at home one week after birth when the patient was two. His father was a puritanical

[1] These case histories will be published in greater detail in a report on the above-mentioned study by Drs. Ham, Alexander, and Carmichael.

man who was harsh and impersonal to hide his own weakness and insecurity. He was apparently demonstrative of affection and fondled his children as long as they were helpless infants but demanded adult behavior as soon as they were able to walk and talk. The mother was depreciated by the father because she had had an illegitimate child in her adolescence (patient's oldest sister) and was married "out of pity" by the patient's father. She was unable to stand up to the father and during the patient's infancy worked in the family store for several years. The father prevented the mother as well as the older sisters from giving the patient much attention. After the patient entered the first grade, his father insisted that no one read him the funny papers any more because he should learn to read for himself. Constant pressure was brought to bear on him to behave like an adult and yet he was continually restricted in the active pursuit of his interests.

The inability to express hostility openly, particularly in respect to sibling rivalry, is present in almost all patients.

E.B., a 24-year-old single colored woman, was a prodigy and progressed rapidly in her school years. She was extremely conscientious, never truant. Her mother was a teacher and "a very intelligent and beautiful woman." The patient was obviously competing with her but never expressed her hostility openly. When her mother became ill, the patient took over the responsibility for her two younger sisters and assumed the function of mother toward them. She supported them financially even during her college years. She has always been self-sufficient and extremely ambitious and has controlled or repressed most of her feminine desires in order to reach her intellectual goals.

The urge toward self-perpetuation through childbearing is clearly shown in another case:

After working her way through high school and college, D.B. gave up her ambition to be a doctor and "settled" for training as a pharmacist. At eighteen she married a childhood friend and they ran a business together. Despite her frigidity she wanted to have children, and in fourteen years she had five children, whom she named Kerry, Barry, Gary, Terry and Mary. She stated that "if my husband hadn't died I would have had all the children that medical science could deliver to me. They are hard to have and so painful, but the more it hurts the more you love them." Since her husband's death, the patient has carried on two jobs simultaneously in order to make sure that the children have sufficient clothing. In addition to this she took a great-aunt into her home who did nothing and had to be taken care of.

The counterphobic mechanism of handling anxiety is illustrated in the following case:

S.K., a 43-year-old white man, was attacked by gunmen. Instead of submitting to their demands he attacked them and was knocked unconscious by a blackjack. For some time following this experience, he had dysphonia and blepharospasm. He maintained that he was never conscious of fear. In several instances when he was either falsely accused or forced to unsafe practices by his foreman, he became enraged and stalked the foreman to his office with an intent to have a fist fight with him.

The strong desire for pregnancy is seen in this case:

F.C., a 36-year-old white married woman, was the oldest of ten siblings, of whom only four survived. She remained at home and helped her mother until she was thirty. Throughout her adolescence and until her marriage at thirty-one she felt great fear in front of men. However, at thirty she became engaged in spite of the father's objections but suffered severe nervousness, had diarrhea, and lost weight during the entire engagement period. She had a strong conscious desire for pregnancy and became pregnant almost immediately after marriage. As soon as she knew she was pregnant she began to feel "wonderful," and during the pregnancy and the first two years after delivery she regained and surpassed her original weight and felt stronger and happier than she had ever been in her life. During this same period she was exposed to continuous insecurity because of housing difficulties that were the common lot of women who followed their enlisted husbands from one army camp to another. Her symptoms began when the patient and her husband went to live in the home of the husband's parents. Further pregnancies became financially out of the question. The patient decided to work and earn money so that they could establish their own home, gain independence and security, and have more children.

Illustrative of the typical dreams about death are the following cases:

D.B. reported dreams which had awakened her with much anxiety. "Grandmother and grandfather were lying in their coffins and reached out in an effort to drag me in; grandmother was dead, covered with flies, and I was trying to brush them off; my husband was either chasing me and trying to catch me or trying to drag me into his coffin." The patient remarked in telling these dreams: "I have always been afraid of death." On a pass from the hospital she wrote her will.

C.D., a 33-year-old colored woman, reported the following dream. "A casket came rolling up to the bed and there was an old white man in it with a beard and he reached for me."

J.K., a 42-year-old white married woman, dreamed frequently of beds. The dreams always occurred before a member of the family died. Once she dreamed of five beds, "mother, father, two children, and husband." A week before the interview she dreamed "I was making a bed. It was mine." She thought this meant that she was going to die.

PSYCHOSOMATIC CONSIDERATIONS

In view of the known stimulating function of the thyroid gland in the growth of the infant, it becomes tempting to relate the hyperactivity of this gland specifically with the apparent need of the hyperthyroid patient to become mature in an accelerated tempo. There can be no question that the patient's constant effort to maintain a pseudo maturity must be quite stressful and may serve to activate the secretion of thyrotropic hormone by the anterior pituitary gland. Consequently, when the psychological defenses against frustrated dependent needs (such as hyperactivity, helping others, or assuming a maternal role) break down and the subject is no longer able to master his underlying anxiety, the stress may become overwhelming and overstimulate that system which regulates the process of maturation and which has been chronically taxed since early infancy because of the constant demand for accelerated maturation and long-range effort.

The ultimate question still remains unanswered: why do these patients react to insecurity with progressive effort toward maturation and not by regressive symptoms? The fact that their dependent tendencies have been consistently thwarted by circumstances alone does not fully explain this type of response. It is possible that they have previously gone through a period of successful adaptation, probably in earliest infancy, which encouraged their tendency toward independence. Heredity, of course, may be a decisive factor.

Most authors recognize, besides environmental influences, a hereditary factor in an inherited susceptibility to hyperthyroidism, but they vary concerning the evaluation of its significance. As experienced a clinician as Moschcowitz, for example, is inclined to stress the importance of environment, while Brown and Gildea emphasize the inherited constitution. Be that as it may, there can be little doubt that the hyperthyroid patient is one who has been trying to maintain a lifelong struggle against his anxiety by attempting to achieve self-sufficiency prematurely and that this pseudo maturity may prove so stressful as to cause a break in balance when the life situation makes the struggle impossible.

Specific Dynamic Pattern in Thyrotoxicosis

Frustration of dependent longings and persistent threat to security (exposure to death and other threatening experiences) in early life ——→ unsuccessful premature attempts to identify with object of dependent cravings ——→ continued effort toward premature self-sufficiency and to help others ——→ failure of strivings for self-sufficiency and taking care of others ——→ thyrotoxicosis.

2. FATIGUE STATES

Fatigue is a subjective response to excessive and prolonged activity. It may appear as physical exhaustion after bodily exertion or as mental fatigue after prolonged intellectual concentration. Emotional participation, interest, and zest are important factors. In performing a tedious routine activity a person may feel fatigued after relatively mild exertion, while he may not experience exhaustion during strenuous work if he is keenly interested in what he is doing.

The precise relationships between such emotional factors and fatigue are still largely unknown. Here only a special form of fatigue will be discussed, which is associated with changes in the regulation of carbohydrate metabolism.

Acute attacks of extreme fatigue and exhaustion accompanied by lightheadedness, cold perspiration, fear of fainting, or a free-floating anxiety have been well known to clinicians as manifestations of hypoglycemia. In several such cases, hyperinsulinism caused by pancreatic adenoma has been found as the underlying factor.

In the last fifteen years spontaneous hypoglycemia has been observed by a number of authors. After the introduction of insulin-shock therapy it became evident that the psychological sequelae of hypoglycemia caused by the injection of insulin were identical with those observed in the spontaneous cases. Functional hyperinsulinism has been assumed, therefore, as the immediate cause. The psychological manifestations in such cases have been described both by psychiatrists and by internists such as Wilder; Rennie and Howard; Romano and Coon; Himwich and others (249, 186, 190, 119). Wilder emphasizes the fact that in addition to the bodily symptoms (fatigue, hunger, perspiration, and tremor), characteristic psychological concomitants are present, such as dullness of consciousness, weakness in concentration, abulia, and a depressive or anxious state of mind. In more serious attacks even mannerisms, changes of speech, double vision, and ataxia (striopallidary symptoms) can be observed. Himwich classifies five definite successive stages which follow as the various regions of the brain become affected in the metabolic derangement:

(1) The cortical phase, with sweating, salivation, muscular relaxation, and tremors, together with a gradual dimming of consciousness.

(2) The subcortico-diencephalic phase, in which the outstanding symptom is motor restlessness manifesting itself in primitive movements such as snarling, grimacing, and grasping.

(3) The mesencephalic phase, characterized by tonic spasm with a positive Babinski reflex.

(4) The premyelencephalic phase, in which the tonic spasms change to extensor spasms. This phase corresponds to the manifestations seen in the decerebrated dog of Sherrington.

(5) The myelencephalic phase, in which a deep coma sets in. In this a parasympathetic tonus is predominant.

In the ordinary cases of functional hypoglycemia usually only the first phase, with weakness, tremulousness, and sweating, can be observed. Anxiety may or may not be present, depending on the patient's personality make-up.

The first psychosomatic study of such cases was carried out by Szondi and Lax in 1929 (231). They studied thirty-one neurotic patients suffering from prostration and apathy who were, according to the customary diagnosis of those days, classified as "neurasthenics." These patients received 50 grams of dextrose by mouth. They showed half as great a rise in blood sugar after half an hour as the twenty-six control cases. This type of blood-sugar curve was called a "flat curve," and a close connection was postulated between the syndrome of fatigue on the one hand and the flat sugar-tolerance curve on the other. They assumed that in neurasthenic individuals the regulatory mechanism of alimentary glycemia is impaired. This flat sugar-tolerance curve is an integral part of the asthenic syndrome.

In 1942, Rennie and Howard reported six patients suffering from "tension depression" who showed similar curves, which became normal after the patients' emotional difficulties were resolved. In 1943, Portis and Zitman (182) observed similar glucose-tolerance curves in forty patients complaining of excessive fatigue; they assumed, as did previous authors, that this might be due to hyperinsulinism caused by an overactivity of the right vagus nerve. They used atropine and eliminated sugar from the diet, allowing only complex carbohydrates. In all cases so treated they observed a return of the blood-sugar curve to normal. These studies gave the first positive indication of the central emotional origin of this condition. Under the influence of these studies, Alexander and Portis (16) undertook a parallel study of nine patients from the psychodynamic point of view. In these cases, the psychodynamic situation was carefully correlated with the state of carbohydrate metabolism. In the reconstruction of the personality development in these patients, an impressive finding was a lack of zest and interest, a complete lack of initiative whether in routine activities, in the office, in school, in study, or in administration of the household. This lack of interest extended into social activities. In most cases, the acute condition of fatigue developed after the patient had to abandon a cherished goal, giving up hope and resigning himself to continue with some distasteful routine against which he revolted internally.

One patient was a 55-year-old woman who suffered from periodic attacks of diarrhea, headaches, and overwhelming fatigue. The patient herself referred to her condition as "pernicious inertia." She dreaded all effort, no matter whether it consisted in household duties, charities, social obligations, or visits to her children. She was caught in a life situation for which there was no solution. This impasse created the inertia.

Another patient, a 37-year-old married businessman, developed fatigue attacks when the main incentive in his work, the guidance and approval of his superiors, ceased, partly because of the slowing down of business and partly because he was promoted to a job which entailed a greater amount of responsibility.

A third patient, a physician, suffered from phobias and developed fatigue attacks after he went into private practice against his own inclination.

An artist developed his attacks immediately after he accepted a position in a business office against which he felt a great emotional resistance. At the same time, he had to give up the career which was his aim in life.

A housewife developed fatigue attacks after her husband refused to have children or to adopt one. Because she had to give up her ardent hope for a child, life became aimless and intolerable for her. She became apathetic and attacks of exhaustion set in.

Alexander and Portis compared this psychological situation with a kind of emotional sitdown strike. Frustrated in their genuine desires and proclivities, being forced to engage in routine activities against their own inclinations, these patients developed their own form of protest. Often this emotional state is accompanied by regressive fantasies and daydreams in which these persons give up all effort and ambition; they indulge only in wishful imagery. The physiological counterpart of this emotional state is characterized by a flat sugar-tolerance curve: a slower and a lesser rise of the blood sugar half an hour after injection than in the normal cases and a lower blood-sugar level after two hours. Like Szondi and Lax, Alexander and Portis found that the original blood-sugar level was not lower than normal. They assumed that there was a causal relationship between the psychological situation and the disturbance of the carbohydrate-regulating mechanisms—i.e., that the disturbance of the carbohydrate metabolism was the physiological counterpart or concomitant of the patient's emotional state.

The working hypothesis advanced by the authors follows Cannon's fundamental views. Preparation for outwardly directed activity stimulated by fear or anger changes the sympathetic-parasympathetic balance in favor of a sympathetic preponderance. They extended Cannon's view in assuming that not only fear and anger but also enthusiasm, zest, and continuous, purposeful striving have a tuning-up effect upon the sympathetic adrenal system. The sympathicotonic effect of zest is probably less intensive but more prolonged than that of fear and rage. Without such an emotional tuning-up of the vegetative functions, sustained effort cannot be carried out with efficiency. It is a well-known fact that a perfunctory activity performed without emotional participation is more fatiguing than extremely strenuous activity carried out with a great amount of emotional participation. It was concluded also that not only is the stimulating effect of sympathetic tonus lacking in these patients, but at the same time under the influence of emotional protest and regression the vegetative functions also regress toward a state of passivity and relaxation characterized by a preponderance of parasympathetic tonus. The organism is then forced either by external pressure or by the internal voice of conscience to undertake continued activity without the necessary sympathetic stimulation. Not only is the sympathetic stimulation absent, but the organism, while exerting itself, is emotionally and vegetatively in a state of regression and relaxation. Physiologically this manifests itself in an increased parasympathetic tonus and increased insulin secretion. The paradoxical situation thus arises that while engaged in effort the organism behaves vegetatively as if it were resting. I called this psychophysiological situation "vegetative retreat." Characteristic of this state is the disturbance of the regulating mechanism of the carbohydrate metabolism.

More recently, the problem of fatigue connected with disturbances of carbohydrate metabolism was further studied by Carlson, McCulloch, and Alexander (44). A comparison was made between 21 patients suffering from fatigue and 29 normal persons with regard to their sugar-tolerance curves. In the fatigue group, the blood-sugar concentration fell farther below the fasting value at the end of the experiment than in the normal group. The difference was statistically significant. Many of the fatigue patients showed a sharp but brief elevation of the blood sugar between 15 and 35 minutes after the injection. Because of these temporary rises, it is inadvisable to place much weight on the 30-minute values. The cause of these sudden temporary rises after an initial drop is not yet fully established. Probably it is the manifestation of a sudden overcorrection in the homeostatic equilibrium and is due to a compensatory sympathetic excitation as a defense measure against the sudden fall of the blood-sugar level which sets in shortly after the injection.

Carlson studied one of the patients in prolonged psychoanalytic consultations, a 31-year-old writer who had suffered from continuous fatigue and acute attacks of exhaustion since he was seventeen. He had gone to college under protest at his father's insistence. Boredom and withdrawal from activities and the fatigue syndrome developed at that time. The feeling of exhaustion, weakness of the legs, and faintness progressively increased. When he forced himself to go out or before he began to work, he often had the feeling of tension, tremors, excessive perspiration, "the jitters." He tried to calm himself by smoking and drinking coffee incessantly.

The patient was an unwanted child, small at birth, and remained slight and physically underdeveloped his whole life. He suffered from inferiority feelings because of his small stature and weakness. The parents' marriage was unhappy; the father drank heavily and neglected and abused his family. All his life the patient remained very close to his sister, who was three years younger than he. He developed a tremendous fear of his father; it stood out in his memory that when his father caught him masturbating, he threatened him with insanity. When he was only eight years old, his father insisted on his working around the house, peddling articles, or caddying, all of which he did only under internal protest. When he was ten, he had a sexual relationship with his sister. To run away with her into "the never-never land" was for a long time a cherished regressive fantasy. In school he gradually withdrew from activities; he was afraid of both teachers and students. He changed colleges several times and at twenty-three started to work in a factory. For a while, he also worked as a sailor and as a day laborer, but finally he began to write and do editorial work, for which he had talent. He was successful and able to do consistent work.

In this patient the "vegetative retreat" can be clearly reconstructed. As a defense against his regressive trend on the one hand and under the external pressure, at first of his father and later of external necessity, the patient drove himself to activity and accomplishment against which he had a deep-seated revulsion. Unconsciously, he identified himself with the easier life of his younger sister, repudiated his masculine obligations, and regressed in his daydreams to a passive, dependent existence. He could not, however, fully accept this retreat, which conflicted with his pride and ambition. Under the influence of this conflict he drove himself to achievement. His hostile competitive attitude toward the father and later toward rivals stirred up anxiety and further prompted him to retreat.

This psychodynamic constellation—the conflict between passive, dependent wishes and reactive aggressive ambition— is widespread, if not universal, in our civilization and can hardly be claimed as a specific explanation of this type of fatigue syndrome. More specific in fatigue cases, apparently, are the following psychodynamic factors:

(1) A lack of hope of achieving some cherished goal; a frustrating struggle against insuperable odds.

(2) A lack of genuine incentive. Activities, mostly routine in nature, are carried out primarily under external pressure or on account of internal compulsion, but not on the basis of an absorbing interest.

(3) The role of anxiety is less constant. In a number of cases the prolonged frustrations create compensatory hostile aggressiveness which leads to anxiety. This further contributes to a regressive retreat from activity.

(4) In a number of male cases there is a conspicuous feminine identification which opposes aggressive ambitious attitudes.

In the case studied by Carlson, the correlation between the emotional states and the changes in the sugar-tolerance curve were well demonstrated. During hospitalization, three curves taken in different emotional states show marked differences. After an initial phase of tension and fatigue the patient showed a disturbed curve; after ten days' stay in the hospital, during which time his tension and fatigue diminished through psychotherapy, a normal curve was obtained. It seems probable that although the fatigue syndrome may in many cases become chronic and characteristic of the patient, nevertheless we are dealing not with a disease entity but with a transitory physiological disturbance. It is probable that everyone grows more fatigued during uninspired or hopeless effort and that this greater fatigability is based on changes in carbohydrate metabolism. To function smoothly during effort, the organism needs the stimulating effect of zest, under the influence of which the regulation of carbohydrate metabolism takes place more efficiently. The organism which is forced to perform against its own will shows not only an emotional protest but also its physiological counterpart, a disturbance in the regulation of mobilization and utilization of carbohydrates.

Many patients can be helped by changing external circumstances, permitting them to pursue their real inclinations. In other cases, internal conflicts do not allow such a simple solution and require systematic psychotherapy.

There is no specific personality type which falls into this category, and to some degree any person may show the temporary symptoms of this type of exhaustion. The use of atropine and of a diet containing no sugar, but only complex carbohydrates, can be of help to combat acute symptoms. It appears that the sudden ingestion of sugar has a beneficial effect of only short duration in counteracting fatigue and often aggravates the symptoms by provoking counter-regulatory homeostatic mechanisms (alimentary hyperinsulinism). This is the rationale of avoiding sugar in the diet and allowing only complex carbohydrates, which do not change the blood-sugar level so suddenly. As discussed before, the beneficial effects of atropine consist in paralyzing the vagus nerve, which is one of the regulators of the internal secretion of the pancreas.

In all cases in which there is a chronic conflict situation, neither dietary and pharmacological measures nor manipulation of the external life situation can achieve more than some temporary relief from the symptoms. Such cases require a consistent psychotherapeutic approach.

3. DIABETES MELLITUS

It is generally acknowledged that psychological factors may influence the course of diabetes mellitus, but the possible etiological significance of such factors has not been established.

That there is a "susceptibility" to the development of diabetes is indicated by the numerous studies which reveal a high familial incidence attributable to the inheritance of one or more genes (Joslin—128). Since the orderly metabolism of the foodstuffs is dependent upon the integrated activity of the intracellular enzymes and their regulation by the endocrine and nervous systems (Soskin and Levine—216), a disturbance in these systems may result in the diabetic syndrome. The susceptible individual is probably born with some limitation of one or another of the regulatory systems and may succumb to a sufficiently intense or prolonged stress. According to Colwell, diabetes actually begins with birth, irrespective of the fact that it may only become clinically apparent much later in life (Colwell—48).

It is generally assumed that diabetes mellitus in man results from an insufficiency of insulin. This insufficiency may be due either to a decrease in the production of insulin by the pancreas or to an increase in the destruction of insulin by the tissues (Mirsky—162). Irrespective of the responsible mechanisms, the end result of the insufficiency is an increase in the rate at which glycogen is converted to sugar and an increase in the mobilization of fats and proteins from their depots to the liver, where they undergo conversion to glucose, acetone bodies, and other intermediary and end products. This results in an impoverishment of the tissues in glycogen, while the blood becomes rich in glucose, and glycosuria ensues.

Cannon demonstrated that fear and anxiety can produce glycosuria in the normal cat and normal human. This supported the hypothesis that emotional stress may produce a disturbance in the carbohydrate metabolism even in the non-diabetic (Cannon—43). However, more recent evidence indicates that although "emotional glycosuria" can be induced in the majority of non-diabetic subjects by intensive emotions, a significant rise in their blood-sugar concentration does not occur at the same time (Mirsky—160). In other words, normal subjects can develop "emotional glycosuria," but they rarely develop "emotional hyperglycemia." Apparently, when the physiological mechanisms responsible for the maintenance of the blood-sugar level are adequate, as in the normal subject, there is a rapid compensation for any emotionally induced change. In the diabetic the regulatory mechanisms are disturbed, and therefore homeostatic equilibration becomes impossible. This explains the widespread observation that emotional upheavals may aggravate the existing metabolic disturbance in the diabetic. It is probable that such aggravation of the diabetic state is due to an increased breakdown of liver glycogen, which in turn can be attributed to an activation of the autonomic nervous system and the secretion of epinephrine. This is in accord with Cannon's emergency concept, and it may be the mechanism responsible for the fluctuations which occur from day to day in the diabetic subject.

It is conceivable that individuals with some limitation of their physiological regulatory mechanisms may develop temporary hyperglycemia under excessive emotional stress. Such individuals undoubtedly have some limitations in their regulation of carbohydrate metabolism, but not of sufficient degree to collapse completely under the particular strain. It is also possible that prolonged and repetitive stress may result in a permanent failure of the relatively inadequate physiological systems, with the result that diabetes mellitus ensues.[1]

Dunbar (75) concluded from her "profile studies" that diabetic patients have greater than normal difficulties in exchanging their infantile dependent state for a more mature independent one. They tend to regress more easily to a dependent attitude and assert their independent strivings mainly in words and little in action. According to her, the diabetic group in general is more passive than active and has a tendency toward masochism and indecisiveness.

In a psychiatric study of diabetic children, Bruch and Hewlett (42) observed that in one-third of their cases the disease

---

[1] The mechanism whereby a chronic psychic tension may induce such failure is offered by Selye's description of the "Adaptation Syndrome." See page 76.

appeared coincident with a disturbance of family relationships, such as divorce, separation, etc. They found that some diabetic children have a tendency to compulsive behavior and submissiveness while others fight back by the way of passive resistance. These authors could find no specific personality type.

The profiles of Dunbar reveal primarily the defense of the patient rather than the conflicts which may be specifically related to the genesis of the disease. The latter can be established by psychoanalysis.

Dunbar reported the analysis of a 29-year-old man who developed diabetes five years after his treatment was interrupted (75). His pattern was similar to that which she found typical of the whole diabetic group. Daniels (55) psychoanalyzed a 33-year-old businessman and concluded that his diabetes could be attributed to chronic anxiety which was associated with unconscious infantile fears of being overpowered and injured because of hostile rebellious and sexual strivings. Meyer, Bollmeier, and Alexander (150) studied two cases, a male and a female, and observed that both patients had unusually strong tendencies to receive and be taken care of. These patients "retained an infantile dependent and demanding attitude and felt frustrated because their demands for attention and love were out of proportion to the reality situation of an adult and consequently were never adequately satisfied. To this frustration the patients reacted with hostility. Diabetes developed when these infantile wishes conflicted with the demands that were frustrated."

Psychoanalytic studies of a large number of patients with diabetes mellitus is now in progress at the Chicago Institute for Psychoanalysis. These studies suggest that "the patient with diabetes mellitus has some basic conflict related to the acquisition of food and that this reflects itself in exaggerated aggressive oral incorporative tendencies. These incorporative impulses manifest themselves in a variety of ways. Thus, there may be a tendency to reject food and subsequently an increased need for replenishment. This need may express itself in an insatiable desire for food, in the wish to be fed, and in excessive demands for receptive gratifications in interpersonal relationships. The incorporative impulses manifest themselves also in an exaggeration of identification with the mother and consequently there may develop an impairment of psychosexual development. In the male, this exaggerated identification with mother leads to an intensification of basic bisexuality. In the female, the hostile identification with the mother activates marked defenses against feminine sexuality, especially with regard to propagative functions" (Benedek, Mirsky, *et al*).[1]

The most important precipitating factor in the genesis of the clinical syndrome of diabetes is obesity, which is present in nearly 75 per cent of the cases. Obesity itself, however, cannot be considered the cause of the diabetes, since only about 5 per cent of obese patients develop diabetes. There is ample evidence that obesity produces an increased demand for insulin. When the pancreatic capacity is adequate, the increased demand for insulin is compensated for. In those obese patients in whom the rate of insulin destruction or utilization is excessive and beyond the capacity of the regulatory mechanism, a relative insulin insufficiency and eventually diabetes will develop. It was indicated in Chapter 9 that overeating is usually the result of some disturbance in the emotional development of the individual. Consequently, psychological factors are etiologically important in those patients who develop diabetes mellitus in consequence of overeating.

On the other hand, the presence of aggressive oral-incorporative tendencies in diabetes may be originally the expression of an inherited physiological deficiency. The potentially diabetic child born with such an anlage can never satisfy his

---

[1] These observations were made in a current investigative work which is in progress in the Institute for Psychoanalysis, Chicago.

biological need. His excessive oral demands may result from this basic physiological insufficiency (Mirsky—159). This phenomenon would be analogous to that observed in the increased appetite for salt in the patient with adrenal cortical insufficiency, or in the self-selection of a high salt intake by the adrenalectomized rat.

The onset of diabetes mellitus, like that of any chronic disease, can produce profound psychological changes in patients as well as in the various members of their family and social groups. Their pride may be hurt, their fears and feelings of inadequacy may become exaggerated, their need to be taken care of by others may become intensified, and their hostility may be stimulated. According to the various forms of defense against these exaggerated tensions, the reaction to the onset of the illness may vary markedly and appear as paranoid depressive and hypochondriacal symptoms. Some patients react with apathy, which may be interpreted as an adaptive behavior aimed at the conservation of energy.

Alexander and his collaborators (150) noted that the glycosuria of their patients increased under the strain of the conflict between their infantile wishes to receive and be taken care of, and the demands to give and to take care of others. Withdrawal from the conflict into self-pity and passivity was associated with a decrease in glycosuria. This observation is in accord with the more recent studies conducted by Benedek, Mirsky, and other members of the Chicago Psychoanalytic Institute, which show a correlation between glycosuria and ketosuria and psychic tension resulting from increased demanding attitudes of the patient, which in turn can be attributed to the frustration of his receptive needs.

Reference has been made to the frequent aggravation of the clinical course of diabetes mellitus by emotional tensions induced by a variety of life situations. This is particularly important in the etiology of diabetic acidosis and coma. This grave complication can be attributed to any factor which will induce an impoverishment of the liver's glycogen depot (Mirsky—161). With an increase in hepatic glycogenolysis the products of fat catabolism, the ketone bodies (aceto-acetic and beta-hydroxybutyric acids), also increase. The secretion of the ketone bodies into the circulation at a rate which exceeds their utilization by the tissues results in ketonemia and ketonuria. The ketone bodies bind base, and this, together with the dehydration and other results of ketosis, favors the development of acidosis and eventually coma.

Anything which stimulates loss of glycogen in the liver can precipitate acidosis, such as starvation, gastrointestinal disturbances, infections, etc. An equally common cause is the omission of insulin (Mirsky—161). From a study of twelve patients who were repeatedly admitted to the hospital in diabetic acidosis, Rosen and Lidz (193) concluded that rather than emotional tension, the willful abandonment of the diabetic regime played a primary role in the etiology of the acidosis. According to these authors, patients with recurrent acidosis utilized their diabetes "as a means of escape into either the shelter of the hospital or through suicide." The studies of Hinkle and Wolf (121) show, however, that emotional tension can induce ketosis even though the patient does adhere to a diabetic regime. They described an anxious, maladjusted girl who developed ketonemia under the influence of fear in a stressful life situation. They demonstrated also that with the experimental continuation of the stress, the ketosis progressed to the stage of clinical acidosis. In another study involving 25 subjects with diabetes mellitus, Hinkle, Conger, and Wolf (120) observed 50 instances of clinical ketosis to occur under emotional conflict. They found that a traumatic interview can cause an elevation of the blood ketones and that this would occur more rapidly in severe diabetes. It would therefore appear that significant emotional conflicts can directly influence the production of ketone bodies. The mechanism whereby this may be achieved has been described above.

Some clinicians believe that it is essential to restrict the diabetic's food intake rigidly so as to render him aglycosuric; others advocate a free diet as long as he remains free from acetonuria and clinical symptoms. The conservative group gives little attention to the fact that a restriction of diet, in terms of calories or grams, means more than a restriction of food; it means frustration and intensifies the insecurity of the diabetic which derives from the realization that he is different from the healthy members of his environment. The physician who imposes a rigid discipline assumes the role of a punitive, rejecting parent and thereby aggravates the patient's existing rebellion and resentment of parental authority. On the other hand, free diet favors obesity and may become just as harmful as is the restricted diet. The permissive attitude of the physician may be interpreted as lack of interest and arouse hostility and guilt, which in turn may unfavorably influence the course of the disease. At the same time, the resulting obesity may further aggravate the physiological derangement.

The physician should be concerned with the amount of calories the patient retains rather than the amount that the patient eats or excretes. The proper use of insulin permits this on a normal diet. At the same time, he must treat the patient as a person rather than merely a caloric apparatus. The diabetic patient will have to become aware of his unconscious demands and his frustrations and make such compromises as are more consistent with both his chronological age and his social milieu. Then he will act and eat as a normal individual and will not harm either himself or his environment.

Chapter XIV

Emotional Factors in the Disturbances of the Joints and Skeletal Muscles

1. RHEUMATOID ARTHRITIS

THE ROLE of emotional factors in the pathogenesis of rheumatoid arthritis has long been suspected and explicitly recognized by a number of clinicians. A conspicuous feature of this disease—its capricious course, its inexplicable remissions and relapses—points to emotional conflicts as partly responsible. Only a few systematic psychosomatic studies have been made on arthritic patients. Although many occasional clinical observations have been published, they are not discussed in this book and the reader is referred to Dunbar's *Emotions and Bodily Changes* (71).

Among the systematic studies, Booth's (34) and Halliday's (113, 114) deserve special mention. Many of their observations have been corroborated by systematic studies carried out in the Chicago Institute for Psychoanalysis by Johnson, Louis Shapiro, and Alexander (126). Since most of the patients studied were women, this discussion deals primarily with female cases. The first feature noted with great regularity is a tendency

toward bodily activity, manifesting itself in a predilection for
outdoor pursuits and competitive sports. This is particularly
outstanding in the pre-adolescent and adolescent age, during which the women patients show decidedly tomboyish
behavior. In adult life these patients show strong control of
all emotional expression. Both Booth and Halliday observed
these personality features. In addition to the tendency to
control their feelings, these patients tend also to control their
human environment, their husbands and children. They are
generally demanding and exacting toward their children and
at the same time worry about them and do a great deal for
them. It is, however, a domineering type of solicitude, a mix-
ture of the tendency to dominate with the masochistic need
to serve other people. This masochism at first glance seems to
be in contradiction to the aggressive domination, but while
they serve their environment and sacrifice themselves for
members of the family, they are also dominating and controlling them.

In their sexual attitude these patients are also strikingly
similar; they show an overt rejection of the feminine role
which is often called in psychoanalytic literature the "masculine protest reaction." They assume certain masculine attitudes; they compete with men and cannot submit to them. It
is interesting that most of these women patients select compliant and passive men as their mates. Several of the husbands
even had physical defects, more than could be easily explained
by coincidence. For the most part, the husbands readily accept
the role of serving their incapacitated wives as the disease
progresses.

On superficial inspection, the precipitating emotional factors seem to be without a common denominator: they cover a
wide range of external events. Indeed, they run the whole
gamut of life situations: birth of a child, miscarriage, death
in the family, change in occupation, sudden change in marital
situation or sexual relationship, a great disappointment in

some interpersonal relationship. It is therefore not astonishing that such an observant investigator as Halliday found little rhyme or reason in precipitating factors.

If, however, we focus our attention on what these various events mean to the patients, we can reduce the precipitating causes to a few significant psychodynamic factors. They appear in three constellations: (1) The disease often begins when an unconscious rebellion and resentment against men has been increased by certain vicissitudes of life; for example, when a patient was abandoned by a man with whom she had felt safe, or when a previously compliant man became more assertive, or when a man in whom the patient had invested a great deal disappointed her. (2) The disease may also be precipitated by events which tend to increase hostility and guilt feelings, previously latent. For example, the birth of a child which reactivates an old sibling rivalry may be the precipitating factor. Guilt may be mobilized when opportunity for sacrifice and service becomes thwarted, as in the event of a miscarriage or of the death of a hated dependent relative or when the patient is forced into a situation where she must accept help beyond her ability to compensate with service. Exacerbation of guilt increases the patient's self-imposed inhibitions and activates hostility which she cannot express because she can no longer combine it with doing service for others. The combination of service and domination which had been the way of expressing hostile impulses in a masked fashion is disrupted. (3) In a few cases the disease was precipitated through sexual experiences at the moment when the patient was forced to accept the feminine role against which she had reacted with an increased masculine protest.

These precipitating events gave us a good starting point for reconstructing the vulnerable spots in the personality structure of these patients. The general psychodynamic background in all cases is a chronic inhibited hostile aggressive state, a rebellion against any form of outside or inside pressure, against being controlled by other persons or against the inhibitory influence of their own hypersensitive consciences. The masculine protest reaction in sexual relations is the most conspicuous manifestation of this rebellion against being dominated.

This central psychodynamic finding, a chronic inhibited hostile rebellious state, could be traced back in most cases to a highly characteristic early family constellation, usually a strong, domineering, demanding mother and commonly a more dependent, compliant father. Booth and Halliday were impressed by this finding. Booth speaks of the stern parents of his patients, and Halliday found that the arthritic patient had at least one domineering parent and that self-restriction began early in life. As little girls our patients developed dependence upon and fear of the cold, aggressive mother and at the same time harbored rebellion which they did not dare express because of this dependence and fear. This inhibited rebellion against the mother is the nucleus of their hostile impulses. It is later transferred to men and to everyone within the family. Subsequently, when they become mothers, they reverse the situation of the past and control their children as they have been controlled by their own mothers.

The following case histories are illustrative: [1]

Mrs. S. G., aged 28 years, developed painful, stiff muscles immediately after she discovered that her husband had had a love affair. After persistent pain and stiffness of the muscles for a few months, she developed arthritis. Her mother was a conscientious but cold woman; the father had deserted the family when the patient was two years old. She was very competitive with an older brother and spent much of her childhood in outdoor activities. She felt that her mother's role, and the position of women in general, was unbearable and said openly she would rather die than tell her husband she loved him, even if she did. "Then I could never be on top." She refused sexual intercourse for

[1] Quoted from A. Johnson, L. B. Shapiro, and F. Alexander: "A Preliminary Report on a Psychosomatic Study of Rheumatoid Arthritis," *Psychosom. Med.* 9:295, 1947.

several months after marriage, had never had an orgasm, and agreed only infrequently to sex relations. Although her husband had been a prize fighter and she was a frail-appearing little woman, she always headed the household and made the decisions, directing her three young daughters in assisting her excellent housekeeping. Her husband's infidelity was the first indication of his rebellion and of her inability to compete with him and control him. When frustrated in her competition the hostility increased, found no outlet and the muscle soreness and arthritis followed. During analysis she consistently refused to go out with him for recreation and finally he was unfaithful to her for the second time. This led to an acute exacerbation of the illness.

Another patient showed conspicuously the masochistic need to serve. She was the 32-year-old mother of three children, the eighth of nine siblings. The following statement gives a succinct picture of her personality: "I am very anxious to get over my arthritis so I can finish having my family. If my mother had not had such a large family, I would never have existed." As a young child she not only did heavy housework and cared for her invalid mother, but she also assisted the father with duties on the farm, although there was a younger brother. All the siblings went to college; after completing high school she went to live with her older sister in order to help care for her many children. In her marriage she continued to display the same slavishly serving attitude toward her three daughters and her husband. Reaction to a miscarriage marked the onset of her arthritic symptoms. On entering analysis she said characteristically, "I have no emotional problems, but I am happy to do anything for science." The emphasis upon being of service to others allowed her to discharge hostile aggressive tendencies without feeling guilty about them.

As a general psychodynamic formulation of precipitating causes and exacerbations, we postulate a predisposing personality factor which develops as the result of excessively restricting parental attitudes. In the little child the most primitive expression of frustration is random motor discharge. If, through punitive measures, this discharge becomes associated with fear and guilt, then in later life whenever fear and guilt arise there results a psychological "strait-jacket." These patients try to achieve an equilibrium between aggressive impulses and control. They learn to discharge aggression through muscular activity in acceptable channels: hard work, sports, gardening, actively heading the house. They also learn to relieve the restrictive influence of the conscience by serving others. Whenever this equilibrium is disturbed by specific events which interrupt the adaptive mode of discharging hostility and relieving guilt, the chronic inhibited aggression leads to increased muscle tonus and in some way to arthritis.

In a small number of the cases studied, specific sexual conflicts were handled by the typical symbolic conversion mechanism. Whether this is superimposed on the same character structure as in the majority of our cases or whether this can serve independently as a precipitating factor is an open question. Our present assumption is that these patients express and discharge their repressed rebellious tendencies through the skeletal muscles by increased muscle tonus. This would put their symptoms in the category of hysterical conversion. At least, the *modus operandi* is the same as in conversion hysteria—namely, the expression of an unconscious conflict by somatic changes in the voluntary muscles. We assume that muscle spasms and increased muscle tonus caused by repressed hostile impulses under certain conditions may precipitate an arthritic attack.

An understanding of the psychodynamics of rheumatoid arthritis throws light upon many of the remissions as well as on the relapses which take place in patients during analysis. If an old avenue of discharge for hostility is opened up again through sudden compliance on the part of the husband, the arthritis has been observed to subside. A woman with a very severe arthritis had to be carried about by her husband. When he died suddenly, she got out of bed, assumed charge of everything, traveled across the country for the funeral, and made an immediate recovery which continued for several months.

The recurrence of arthritis when opportunities for masochistic service are diminished has been observed, followed by its subsidence when self-sacrifice is again demanded by family conditions. As patients become more able to receive help under the influence of psychoanalysis, the disease diminishes.

In the study of arthritis one must bear in mind the fact that the personality picture of advanced crippled cases is overlaid by a chronic psychological adaptation of the personality to the state of being crippled. Naturally, the pre-existing character has an influence on the behavior, but new features dominate the picture. Most authors who have studied such cases were impressed by the secondary features, such as stoicism and optimism. In addition to the self-deceptive wish fulfillment, this type of adaptation can be understood by the fact that the diseased condition relieves the patient from guilt feelings and gives him the right to expect attention that was previously withheld or unacceptable. This was clearly seen in a patient who had had to care for a demanding father for years. When her arthritis became advanced she said, "Now he will have to take care of me."

The view that increased muscle tonus is involved in this disease is further substantiated by the extremely common observation that arthritic patients complain of muscular rigidity and tenseness upon awakening. Some of them report sleeping in overflexed positions. In many cases muscular stiffness and pain were the precursors of the first arthritic attack. We may refer to the common use of neostigmine by clinicians who believe relief of muscle spasm and pain can occur even in a burned-out joint.

I wish to emphasize that at the present state of our studies we are not yet able to evaluate the etiological significance of all of these findings. We surmise that inhibited hostile impulses lead to increased muscle tension. The hostile impulses seek discharge by muscle contractions, but their inhibition leads to simultaneous increase of the tonus in the antagonist muscles. This simultaneous activation of antagonists may traumatize the joints and favor an already existing disease process which perhaps has a yet unknown somatic basis.

The propensity of the arthritic patients to express repressed tendencies through skeletal muscles was well demonstrated by French and Shapiro in their study of the dreams of a patient suffering from rheumatoid arthritis (91).

Male patients also show a chronic state of inhibited rebellious hostility. This seems to be a reaction against unconscious dependent feminine trends for which they overcompensate with aggressiveness. The inhibition of these aggressive impulses creates a psychodynamic picture similar to that seen in female patients.

The final validation of these concepts will have to wait until extensive myographic studies have measured the changes in muscle tension in arthritic and nonarthritic patients in correlation with various emotional states. The preliminary results of a jointly conducted study by the Psychosomatic Institute of the Michael Reese Hospital and the Chicago Institute for Psychoanalysis show that a greater than normal degree of muscular response to emotional stimuli is present in arthritic patients and in some other patients, such as hypertensives. This indicates that still further factors will be found which characterize the arthritic patient. At the present state of our knowledge, it is still too early to draw any conclusions as to the effect of psychotherapy in these cases. In evaluating the fact that many of these patients have been successfully treated by psychotherapy, one must bear in mind the frequency of spontaneous remissions of shorter or longer duration in this disease.

Specific Dynamic Pattern in Rheumatoid Arthritis

Restrictive and (*in women*) overprotective parental influence in infancy ⟶ rebellion against restrictive parental influences ⟶ anxiety ⟶ repression of rebellious tendencies

due to excessive dependence nurtured by parental overpro-
tection ⟶ expression of rebellion in competitive sports and
outdoor activities in childhood and early adolescence ⟶
expression of hostility in combination of serving and controlling environment (benevolent tyranny) in later life; also rejection of feminine role (masculine protest) ⟶ interruption of successful pattern of serving and at the same time dominating the environment ⟶ increase of muscle tonus ⟶
arthritis.

2. THE ACCIDENT-PRONE INDIVIDUAL

The contention of modern psychiatry that most accidents
are not accidents at all but are caused largely by the victim's
own disposition is but a confirmation of common observation.
Strictly speaking, an accident is an occurrence the cause of
which is outside a person's control. A brick falling on a pedestrian's head is a completely accidental event, particularly if
the pedestrian is not warned by a sign that such an event is
likely to occur at a particular place. Most industrial, traffic,
and home accidents, however, are of a different nature. The
sufferer from the accident has some active part in its causation. It is popularly assumed that he was clumsy, tired, absent-
minded, otherwise he might have avoided the accident.

Scientific scrutiny, however, has established that most accidents are not due to such simple human qualities. Certain
people are prone to have more accidents than others, not because they are clumsy or absent-minded, but because of the
total structure of their personality. The significant factor is
not a particular isolated feature such as slow reaction or lack
of intelligence but something much more basic which per-
tains to the totality of the person as an individual. Here are a
few startling facts concerning the human factor in accidents.

More than twenty years ago, Marbe (146), a German psychologist, made the remarkable observation that the person

who has had one accident is more likely to have another one than the person who has never suffered an accident. Statistical studies in large industrial companies have shown that accidents are not evenly distributed among the employees, but that a very small percentage of employees has a very high percentage of the accidents. One might conclude from this that possibly the employees who have the most accidents are those whose assignments are most dangerous. That this is not so, however, is demonstrated by the fact that those persons who have the most accidents in one kind of job also have the most accidents in other jobs. Moreover, those employees who have the worst accident records while on jobs also have the most frequent accidents at home or on the way to work.

In a study of motor-vehicle accidents in Connecticut, it was established that over a six-year period as few as 3.9 per cent of the drivers involved in accidents had as many as 36.4 per cent of all of the accidents (171).

One large company which employs a great number of truck drivers became concerned about the high cost of its automobile accidents and tried to analyze the causes of accidents in order to reduce the frequency. Among other procedures, they examined the accident records of each driver, and finally they transferred those who had the most accidents to other occupations. By this simple device they succeeded in reducing the accident rate to ⅕ of its original level. The most interesting fact in this study is that the drivers who had a high accident rate retained their accident habit in their new occupations. This shows irrefutably that there exists an accident-prone person and that accident-prone individuals are accident-prone in any occupation and in everyday life.

The next problem was to determine those qualities in a person which make him inclined to have accidents. Dunbar (72, 75), who studied a large number of fracture patients with modern methods of psychiatry, describes the accident-prone person as follows: He is decisive or even impulsive; he concentrates upon immediate pleasures and satisfactions. He is apt to act upon the spur of the moment. He likes excitement and adventure, and does not like to plan and prepare for the future. A large number of persons with the accident habit have had a strict upbringing and have derived from this an unusual amount of resentment against persons in authority. Briefly, they are men of action, not of planning, persons who do not interpolate much deliberation and hesitation between impulses and their execution. This impetuousness may have various reasons, but apparently rebellion against restrictions by authority and all form of external coercion is its most common origin. The accident-prone person is essentially a rebel; he cannot tolerate even self-discipline. He rebels not only against external authorities but against the rule of his own reason and self-control.

Intensive psychoanalytic study of a few cases has allowed an even deeper insight into the intricacies of the emotional life of the accident-prone person. Particularly revealing were studies which scrutinized the emotional state of the person immediately before his accident. Dunbar (72, 75); Karl Menninger (153); Rawson (6); Ackerman and Chidester (185); and others have shown that in most accidents there is an element of intention, though intention is by no means conscious. In other words, most accidents are unconsciously motivated. They belong to that category of phenomena which were described by Freud as the errors of everyday life, such as misplacing an object, forgetting to mail a letter, misspelling or mispronouncing a word. Freud showed that such errors are not accidental in the strict sense of the word but are unconsciously intended. When a presiding officer erroneously declared a meeting closed instead of opening it, he had some good but hidden reason for having the meeting over with before it started. A person who carries a letter in his pocket for days has some definite, although unconscious, reason for not mailing it. Most accidents are similarly caused by unconscious motivations, although they usually are of much graver consequence than these harmless errors of everyday life.

Psychoanalytic investigation has revealed the nature of the unconscious motives which induce people to act in a way which invites accidents. The most common motive is a sense of guilt which the victim tries to expiate by self-imposed punishment. The unconsciously induced accident serves this purpose. Since this may sound improbable, I shall try to illustrate it with a few brief examples. Ackerman quotes the following case:

A youth was driving his mother on a shopping tour. He begged her for the use of the car for a fishing party the following day. She refused, whereupon he fidgeted angrily, "accidentally" stepped on the accelerator, and sent the car into a ditch, injuring both himself and his mother.[1]

The combination of revenge and guilt was obvious in this case; the young man punished his mother, but at the same time he punished himself as well.

According to Rawson 60 per cent of patients with fractures studied psychiatrically confessed guilt and resentment in their relationship to some person in connection with the accident. He gives the following examples:

A 16-year-old Puerto Rican said: "It was really my fault because Mother said supper was ready and I was not to go out. I went out anyway, got into a wrestling match and got my arm broken. Anyway, I guess Mother's sorry she's so strict with me."

A 27-year-old woman was hurt sliding down a banister. She had always worked off annoyances with her parents and later with her husband by such tricks. "Perhaps I ought to know better but I wouldn't have been like that if they had had more sense, and had treated me more like a person instead of being so strict."

A secretary fell and fractured her hip. "I asked my friends

[1] N. W. Ackerman and L. Chidester: " 'Accidental' Self-Injury in Children," *Arch. Pediat.* 53:711, 1936.

why I must be punished so. I can't remember ever having done anything wrong, but I must have done something terrible." [1]

The basis of this strange combination of emotions is a deeply ingrained attitude prevalent in our present civilization, that suffering expiates guilt. If the child does something wrong, he is punished. Through the suffering caused by the punishment he makes up for his guilt, and thus deserves and regains the love of his parents. Our criminal laws are based on the same attitude. The offender serves his punishment, after which he can return to the community as a free person, having expiated for his wrongdoing. The human conscience applies this same principle within the personality, acting as an internalized judge who demands suffering for our wrongdoings. Suffering relieves the pangs of guilty conscience and restores the inner peace.

The most common cause of guilt feelings in children is hostile, rebellious impulses against the parents. The accident-prone person retains his childhood rebellion against persons in authority even in his later life; and he also retains the guilt reactions originally felt toward his parents. The combination of these two, resentment and guilt, is a common factor in accidents. Those people who have a great deal of this self-punitive urge constitute the majority of accident-prone individuals. The guilt feelings are convincingly revealed in the frequent question of the sufferer right after his accident; "Why did it happen to me? What did I do to deserve it?" These questions show that the guilt feeling, although not quite conscious, is vaguely sensed by the patient.

More than twenty years ago I became convinced of the unconsciously intended nature of certain accidents. I was consulted by an intelligent man in middle life suffering from a severe depression which had developed out of an unsuccessful struggle for existence. He came from a well-to-do, socially prominent family but had married into a different social stra-

[1] A. T. Rawson: "Accident Proneness," *Psychosom. Med.* 6:88, 1944.

tum. After this alliance his father and family refused to have anything more to do with him. His long struggle for a livelihood terminated (on account of neurotically determined inhibitions) in a total psychic collapse. I advised him to begin an analysis with a colleague, because I had personal relations with him and his family and was well acquainted with his previous history. He found decision difficult. One evening when the final decision was to be made, he asked to visit me, in order to talk over the pros and cons once more. But he did not arrive; he had been run over by an auto in the neighborhood of my home. He was taken to a hospital suffering from severe injuries. It was only the following day that I heard of the accident. When I discovered him in the third-class division of the hospital, he was bandaged up like a mummy. He could not move, and all one could see of his face was his eyes, shining with a euphoric light. He was in good spirits, free from the oppressive melancholy of recent days. The first words with which he greeted me were, "Now I have paid for everything; now I will at last tell my father what I think of him." He wanted to dictate a determined letter to his father immediately, demanding his share of his mother's estate. He was full of plans and was thinking of starting a new life.

What is most impressive in this story is the emotional relief which this patient gleaned from his injury. It freed him from the pressure of his guilty conscience, which was stirred up by his extremely hostile feelings against his family, who refused to recognize his marriage. After the injury he was ready to express freely all his resentment and tell his father what he thought of him.

Occasionally there are other unconscious motives at work in the causation of accidents, such as the wish to avoid responsibility, the wish to be taken care of, even the desire for monetary compensation.

In summary, the accident-prone individual is an impetuous person who immediately converts his momentary impulses into action. He harbors a deeply ingrained rebellion against the excessive regulations of his upbringing—a deep resentment against persons in authority. At the same time he has a strict conscience which makes him feel guilty for this rebellion. In the unconsciously provoked accident he expresses his resentment and revenge, atoning for his rebellion by his injury.

Since the major factors in accidents are not external, such as defective machinery or unfavorable conditions like weather, darkness, etc., but lie in the person who has the accident, the primary measures toward prevention must be directed toward the person himself. There are only two effective ways to approach this human factor: one is to change the individual and the other, to take the accident-prone person away from those occupations where the danger is great. Both measures require reliable methods by which the accident-prone individual can be spotted. Because the psychological factors which predispose an individual to accidents are not simple isolated qualities, they cannot be detected by the usual methods of psychological testing. The psychiatric interview, conducted by an expert, which reveals the whole previous life history of a person is the most reliable method. The accident habit develops early in life and manifests itself in the youngster, in a noticeable inclination to contract physical injuries, even if only minor ones. The combination of excessive resentment and guilt manifests itself in early childhood in various ways familiar to the trained psychiatrist.

Chapter XV

The Functions of the Sexual Apparatus and Their Disturbances

THERESE BENEDEK, M.D.

THE PSYCHOSOMATIC approach to medicine meets its most promising challenge in investigations related to the functions of the sexual apparatus, for in no other field is the relationship between the psychological and the physiological aspects of a function so intimate as in sexuality.

It has been known since time immemorial that the sexual glands—the testes and the ovaries—exert a significant influence on temperament and behavior. Castration, the removal of the testes, as well as spaying, the removal of the ovaries, has always been employed on the farm to achieve temperamental changes useful in the domestication of animals, and to achieve metabolic changes which make their meat more desirable. In the human, too, it has been observed that castration reduces virility, not only because it leads to sterility, but because it is followed by bodily changes in the sex characteristics and by emotional changes which reduce the tendencies toward masculine activities. In a similar way in women, the early removal of the ovaries, or their innate insufficiency, causes sterility and interferes with the development of the physical and emotional female characteristics.

Spectacular experiments around the turn of the century established the role of the sexual glands (gonads) in the production of the sexual hormones. Freud's early assumption that "the disturbed chemistry of the (sexually) unsatisfied person produces anxiety and thus leads to other symptoms" (92) was in accord with the expectation of other biologists of his time. In his first comprehensive study of the theory of sexuality (94), Freud expressed the hope that endocrinology would hold the answer to the problems of normal and abnormal sexual behavior. Since then psychoanalysis has elaborated in great detail the role which sexual drive and its concomitant psychic energy—libido—plays in the dynamics of psychic processes. It has established that the maturation of the sexual function and the integration of the personality are closely interwoven processes. But the endocrinological substratum of sexuality was not included in these investigations. Endocrinology went its own way.

After isolation and synthesis of the steroid hormones, experiments on lower mammals seemed to affirm the thesis that sexual behavior is under simple chemical control. It was established that in lower mammals the cyclical function of the ovaries governs sexual behavior: mating occurs at the height of the periodically recurring *estrus*—heat—which manifests itself in various recognizable activities leading to copulation. Observations in the primates, however, reveal discrepancies in the proportionate relationship between gonad function and mating behavior (Maslow—149). Primates may be stimulated to sexual activity by a variety of factors independent of estrus. In man, the complex and variable stimuli which motivate sexual behavior may conceal the physiological cycle almost completely. When it became evident that sexual behavior could not be explained simply in terms of gonad function, the role of the hormones in the hierarchy and in the interaction of the factors which motivate sexual behavior had to be studied.

From the large body of physiological information we shall cite the bare facts pertinent to the sexual function of all mammals. In both sexes, the gonads are under the regulation of the pituitary gland. Through specific hormones the pituitary influences body growth as well as many aspects of metabolism, and through its *gonadotropic hormones* it stimulates the maturation and controls the functions of the testes and ovaries. The process is simpler in the male than in the female. Under the influence of gonadotropic hormones, the testes produce the male gametes, the *spermatozoa*, and one group of hormones, the *androgens*,[1] which are held to be responsible for the physical and emotional characteristics of virility. In the female, the process is more complex: there is a reciprocal interaction between pituitary function and the ovaries which effects a rhythmical change in the production of gonadotropins, and this, in turn, effects the cyclic nature of the ovarian activity. The ovaries yield the female gametes—*ova*—and two groups of hormones, which are produced in sequence: *estrogens,* which stimulate the maturation of the sex cells, and *progestins,* which secure the nidation and maintenance of the fertilized ova. Both types of hormones have a specific influence upon the secondary sex characteristics and upon the emotional household of woman.

It is established that gonadal hormones are absolutely necessary for the completion of the maturational processes which lead to procreation. However, "the hormone is to be regarded not as a stimulus to behavior, nor as an organizer of the overt response, but merely as a facilitating agent, which increases the reactivity of the specific neuromuscular system to stimula-

[1] The chemical agent of androgens is *testosterone.*

tion." [1] The physiological role of the gonad hormones in the organism is influenced by "a genetically determined responsiveness of the nervous mechanism" (Beach—24). In man, the primary disposition of the nervous system to respond to internal and external stimulation becomes highly complicated by external (cultural) factors which modify the stimuli as well as the responses of the individual to them. Therefore, the effects of the gonad function in an individual can hardly be separated from the psychological factors which determine the development of the personality as a continuous, functioning unity.

A review of the psychoanalytic concepts of personality development, which includes the integration of the normal procreative function with all other functions of the personality, does not belong in the scope of this presentation.[2] In order to elucidate the factors which lead to dysfunctions of the sexual apparatus, the role of emotional bisexuality in the psychosexual maturation will be discussed.

The *sex* of the individual is determined at conception by the chromosome make-up of the gametes. Through this, the embryo is endowed with a potentiality of developing toward one sex. There is evidence, however, that this development is not completely secure; that already in utero, conditions may occur which interfere with the development of the male embryo toward maleness. This occurs, for example, with the inundation of the male embryo with female sex hormones to such a degree that a "sex intergrade" develops. Thus, not the genes but "external" hormonal conditions may account for a

[1] F. A. Beach: *Hormones and Behavior.* New York and London, Paul B. Hoeber, Inc., 1948.

[2] Its most significant dynamic concepts are discussed in F. Alexander's *Fundamentals of Psychoanalysis* (8). A comprehensive presentation of the personality development written by the author of this chapter will appear in *Dynamic Psychiatry*, by Alexander, *et al.*

varying degree of *bisexuality* at birth (Hoskins—122). The
term "bisexuality" refers here not to anatomical hermaphro-
ditism or other manifest forms of "sex intergrades," but to a
*specific predisposition for certain reactions to environmental
influences.* The environment of the new-born is defined
by the still existing symbiosis between mother and child.
Through lactation and physical care, the mother conveys influences which have different significance for the infants of
the two sexes. The hormones which the girl receives from the
mother as well as the developmental tendencies for identification with her are in the direction of the goal of the girl's
later psychosexual development. The boy, however, receives
an endocrine influence through lactation which may intensify
the feminine component in him; the development of the boy
during the oral-receptive phase proceeds through identification with the mother; and this, too, may add to the tendency
toward bisexual reactions, which are in opposition to the goal
of the psychosexual development of men.

The manifestations of psychic bisexuality can be recognized in the early pregenital phases of development. The two-
year-old boy, if he is a "real boy," shows a tendency for self-
assertion and independence, while the "sissy" is afraid of any
new step and recoils from self-assertion in order to assure his
continued dependence on the mother. It is not known
whether endocrine factors play a role in such phenomena.
Children of both sexes produce small amounts of estrogens
and androgens; it is not known, however, whether these hormones participate in the "surplus excitation" which produces
pregenital libido (Alexander—8). Neither is it known
whether there is any change in the "gonad" hormones when
the child enters the *oedipal phase* and turns his erotically
colored demands toward the parent of the other sex and by
this means becomes "guilty" and afraid of punishment from
the parent of the same sex. It seems beyond doubt, however,
that the psychodynamic result of this crucial conflict is

strongly influenced by the bisexual components of the psychosexual anlage. The "emotional reality" of the *castration complex* is only partially dependent upon the intensity of the instinctual wish; it is just as dependent, or more so, upon the environment: upon the punitiveness and seductiveness of the parents, upon the child's security with them; last but not least, it is dependent upon the child's disposition, which makes him experience as a psychic reality the idea that castration, the loss of the penis, is possible. (Alexander and Staercke pointed out that the little boy is prepared for the loss of the penis by such early sensations as the loss of the nipple from the mouth and the loss of the feces from the anus, since he once considered these a part of his self. In the same way, the fleeting sensations of erections, which come and go without his control, may frighten the child.) Psychoanalysis usually reveals that the discovery of the female genital region is the trauma which fixates in the mind of the little boy the idea that the penis can be lost, since there are human beings without it. To him, therefore, the female genitalia may appear as a devouring organ which may incorporate the penis and keep it. Identification with the dangerous individual is the most efficient defense against this fear. Through identification with the mother, the boy develops the *"negative oedipus complex";* instead of identifying himself with his father in the tendency to love the mother, he wants to be loved by the father and wants to replace the mother with him. Such a solution of the oedipus conflict has great value for the emotional economy: it reduces the fear of the female genitals and it also postpones the fear of the father's punishment. The process is similar in girls with strong tendencies toward masculine identification. Such a girl, after she has experienced heterosexual impulses and thus gained the impression that the penis is a "dangerous organ," resolves the oedipal conflict by identifying herself with the father. Through the intense wish to have a penis or by the illusion that she has or will grow one, the girl represses the fear of the male genitals, and at the same time she develops the hope that she is loved by the mother in the same way as the father and/or the brother.

The manifestations of bisexual tendencies may be recognized during the pregenital phases in the variations of the child's identifications. It takes, however, the struggle of the oedipal phase to reveal the quantitative differences between masculine and feminine inclinations, between readiness to take the risks of heterosexual development and the tendency to recoil from it because of the strength of the opposing tendencies. Margaret Gerard in her extensive study on enuresis (99) points out that enuresis, as a neurotic symptom, is the manifestation of a bisexual tendency. Both boys and girls suffer from night terror, the content of which is the fear of being attacked by an adult of the opposite sex. The fear mobilizes the sado-masochistic excitation which is discharged by urination. The behavior of the boys is regressed, passive, and self-deprecatory; the girls are overcompensatorily active, motivated by their masculine identification. From the many possible variations of the oedipus conflict constellations, we have selected one which, because it enhances in the boy the feminine and in the girl the masculine inclinations, reinforces the bisexual tendencies of the individual.

The fixation of the developmental potentialities in a particular direction is one effect of the oedipal phase of development; another result is a new structuralization of the personality, which Freud termed the *superego*. This psychic institution represents the incorporation of the prohibitions which, in our culture, demand the repression of sexual activities in childhood. Through the controlling influence of the superego, the psychological factors gain weight in directing the process of sexual maturation.

The psychic equilibrium is a balance of functions in the various structures of the personality. Accordingly, it depends upon the strength of the ego—its capacity to repress the disturbing stimuli—on the one hand and upon the intensity of the stimuli on the other, whether the *latency period,* a period without awareness of sexuality, develops after the oedipal tendencies have been repressed. There are civilizations in which a latency period is not a cultural requirement. Yet there, too, society develops means and regulations to protect the children from their own and from adults' sexuality (Mead —151). In spite of the strict demands for repression of sexual impulses, there are many children who, during the age of latency (between six and eleven or twelve years), are disturbed by sexual fantasies and activities which lead to conflicts with their environment as well as with their superego. In evaluating the factors which may be responsible for the sexual stimulation of the latency period, one may consider various possibilities: (1) An unqualified surplus excitation is channelized through the sexual apparatus; (2) irrepressible sexual stimuli are due to specific endocrine stimulation; (3) the ego's capacity to suppress sexual impulses is too weak and therefore the not-too-strong instinctual impulses may pass the barrier and request immediate gratification. Analysis may reveal a combination of the factors. It often occurs that the ego appears weak in suppressing the sexual impulses which originate in conflicting tendencies. On the basis of the psychoanalytic evaluation of the individual's development, one may appreciate the role which the sexual experiences of the oedipal and latency periods have played in modifying, precipitating, and/or arresting the psychosexual maturation. But there are no evidences of corresponding deviations in the processes of the endocrine apparatus. Psychoanalytic observations tend to prove that fixations on pregenital levels of sexuality, and their compulsive repetition during the latency period, as well as the castration fear which accompanies or motivates them, delay rather than accelerate the completion of sexual maturation. Fenichel assumed that "every fixation necessarily changes the hormonal status" (83). This assumption could probably not be validated even if the methods of endocrinological investigation were more refined.

At *puberty*, the gonadotropic hormones of the pituitary gland stimulate the production of androgens and of the ovarian hormones, causing, in both sexes, the gradual appearance of the secondary sex characteristics. Puberty—the physiological maturation of the gonads—sets in motion the involved emotional processes of development which constitute the period of *adolescence*. The disquieting symptoms of adolescence represent the manifestations of a reorganization within the personality. This is set in motion by the upsurging "surplus energy" produced by the activities of the gonads and of other growth processes. It would be, however, an oversimplification to assume that during adolescence a physiologically mature sexuality struggles against the inhibitions which, originating in the introjected sexual prohibitions of the past and the sociological realities of the present, may delay sexual gratification. Recent studies of various South Sea people (Montagu—167) have revealed that a period of sterility exists during adolescence in women. This indicates that the completion of physiological maturation takes a long time even in civilizations in which the psychosexual development does not pass through periods of repression and latency. It is simple to expect that the period of adolescence (and the completion of the physiological maturity) takes even longer in our civilization, where the goal of sexual maturation can be achieved only through the reconçiliation of the sexual drive with all other functions of the personality.

During adolescence sexuality changes from a general, pleasurable excitation to an essential need; its ideal satisfaction is achieved only by coitus with a member of the other sex. The upsurging sexual energy, however, stirs up the conflicts of previous developmental periods and their concomitant affects. It recharges the channels of pregenital gratifications and rekindles the anxieties which have accompanied the oedipal conflict. Thus, at the onset of adolescence, a deep-rooted anxiety separates the sexes. The severity of the adolescent conflict, in both sexes, is determined by its two psychodynamic components: the intensity of the instinctual need produced by physiological stimulation; and castration fear, which, rooted in the previous developmental conflicts, is mobilized anew by the physiological stimulation. The adolescent process is an intricate interaction between physiological and psychic forces, which normally leads to the resolution of the castration fear.

Sexual maturity means that the individual has learned to find gratification for his instinctual need in the framework of his conscience. This, even without any further elaboration of the dynamic processes, indicates that genital sexuality in the human adult is under the control of a highly structuralized ego. The genital sexual energy, on its way to achieving gratification, has to comply with conditions determined by the superego and has to overcome resistances set before it by the ego; both the restrictions of the superego and the defenses of the ego may deter and delay the free expression and the discharge of libido. However, not only the ego and superego, but also the instinctual drives may present obstacles to the integration of sexual maturity: fixations on pregenital patterns of gratification may absorb sexual energy; anxiety, produced by pregenital conflicts, may deflect this energy and force it into infantile channels. Thus psychosexual energy may be completely or partially spent in intrapsychic processes. According to such considerations of the economy of intrapsychic processes, it appears that not the production of sexual energy but its spending accounts for the variations in sexual behavior in men.

Even a sketchy presentation of the interaction between sexual maturation and the development of the personality indicates that the integration of the sexual drive from its pregenital sources to genital maturity is the axis around which the organization of the personality takes place. Looking at it from the point of view of sexual function, the sexual drive is organized differently in male and female in order to supply the motivation for their specific functions in procreation.

1. SEXUAL FUNCTIONS OF THE MALE

The male sexual function is performed in a single act: in coitus. The man gratifies his active heterosexual need by this act and, at the same time, discharges the spermatozoa into the female genital canal and thus makes fertilization (conception) possible. The male sexual drive, accordingly, is under the control of one group of sexual hormones—androgens. In the adult, there is a correlation between the gonad hormone production and the urgency of sexual impulses (Pratt—183). However, there is no regularly returning cycle of recessions and reintegrations of the psychosexual pattern comparable directly with the sexual cycle in women. One may observe in men emotional fluctuations which, although they do not occur with regular periodicity, appear to be dependent upon gonadal function. Their manifestations are clinically similar to a light depression. The psychoanalytic material reveals a change in the heterosexual tendency: the general extraverted activities, as well as the sexual desire, appear diminished; the psychosexual energy, concentrated upon the self, brings about a hypochondriacal mood. While in women such an emotional state may be considered as corresponding to low gonadal hormone level, in men the state of the corresponding gonadal hormone production has not been investigated. The tendency to such emotional fluctuations in men may be independent of the gonadal hormone production.

Whatever role the gonadal hormones play in producing and channelizing the genital sexual energy, there are observations which indicate that the end-organs of sexual functions may be stimulated by other than gonadal factors. In this respect, we may regard the perception of libido as the function of the psychic end-organ. Normally, libido is perceived as lust, as a pleasurable drive which, conveyed to the sex organs, sensitizes them to discharge the libidinal tension in satisfactory acts. In a recent paper W. H. Perloff (179) described a case of a eunochoid male who felt heterosexual urges and was able to achieve erection and orgasm. This case, as well as a similar case of a girl with ovarian agenesis who felt normal heterosexual attraction toward men, is unusual. But such cases indicate that in the human, libido and potency may be present although the gonadal hormones are diminished or absent. Other, not unusual, conditions, such as the hypersexuality of post-climacteric individuals, demonstrate also that libidinal tension is not proportionate to gonadal hormone production. On the other hand, there are disparities in libidinous feelings as well as in sexual behavior which cannot be related to the quantities of gonadal hormone production measurable by the present techniques of investigation. The economy of intrapsychic processes—as discussed before—offers explanations for these phenomena. Since the psychosexual energy may be spent in intrapsychic processes, it is readily understandable that the genital sexual energy, although it may result from normal gonadal function, does not reach in every instance the effectiveness which is necessary for the integration of the psychic and somatic aspects of sexuality.

2. SEXUAL FUNCTIONS OF THE FEMALE

In woman, the ebb and flow of the gonadal hormone production renders the interaction between endocrine functions and psychodynamic processes accessible for study. The first of such investigations was attempted when the author, in collaboration with B. B. Rubenstein, studied the psychosexual manifestations of the ovarian functions (28). On the basis of daily temperature charts and vaginal smears, the state of the ovarian cycle was established in a group of women who were undergoing psychoanalysis. The psychoanalytic records were analyzed in an attempt to ascertain whether there are changes and fluctuations in the psychosexual manifestations of the patients, specifically in relation to the ovarian cycle. On the basis of such study, a chart of the menstrual cycle was outlined. When the data, achieved independently, were compared, it was found that they almost exactly coincided; both methods were able to establish the significant phases of the ovarian functions. Sexual behavior in women is motivated by a great variety of factors; the biological tendencies are disguised and modified by cultural patterns and by the developmental processes which determine the individual variations in sexual expression. In spite of the complex psychological structure of human personality, this study established that (1) the emotional manifestations of the sexual drive, like the reproductive function itself, are stimulated by gonad hormones; (2) parallel with the production of estrogen, an active, extraverted heterosexual tendency motivates the behavior; (3) parallel with the progestin phase, the psychosexual energy is directed inwardly as a passive-receptive and retentive tendency; thus (4) parallel with the hormonal cycle, an emotional cycle evolves. The hormonal and emotional cycle together represent the *sexual cycle*.

The sexual cycle begins with the follicular ripening phase, during which estrogens are gradually produced. The active heterosexual tendencies can be recognized in overt or disguised sexual behavior, in dreams and fantasies, and in an increased alertness in the extraverted activities of the individual. Indeed, it appears that estrogens in humans, as in lower mammals, serve to bring about sexual activity. At the same time, estrogens also stimulate the ego to higher integration and co-ordination of its activities in other than sexual areas.[1]

[1] In evaluating the intensity of the heterosexual need, one has to con-

About the time of ovulation, estrogen production reaches its height and merges with the incipient output of progestins; this continuation is the stimulus for the highest level of psychosexual integration, i.e., the biological and emotional readiness for conception. This finds expression in the enhanced libidinal readiness for receiving the mate, or, if this is thwarted, in an increasing emotional tension; this often characterizes the preovulative stage.

After ovulation occurs, the heterosexual tension is suddenly relieved and a period of relaxation follows; the direction of the psychosexual energy changes and becomes concentrated on the woman's body and its welfare. The effect is a generalized erotization; the readiness to receive the sexual partner is usually conscious; the desire for impregnation and for pregnancy is, as a rule, recognizable only in dreams and fantasies. While the activity of the corpus luteum (progestin production) increases, a period comparable to the "quiet period" in lower mammals develops and lasts for several days. The psychological material corresponding to this period might be summarized as preparation for motherhood. This may be expressed as a wish for or a fear of pregnancy and/or a hostile defensiveness against it. Analysis of this material usually reveals the repetition of the conflicts which the woman had in her childhood and which she may unconsciously maintain with her mother; one recognizes the striving for resolution of such conflicts and for reconciliation with the mother, especially in the acceptance of and desire for motherhood. In these cases, fantasies about having children and concern for child care are prevalent in the psychological material. If this

---

sider the changes in affects occurring after its gratification or on account of its frustration; in the latter situation, the emotional tension increases; in the former, it relaxes. In the same way, one must consider the defenses against the heterosexual tendencies in inhibited individuals. In such persons, in coordination with estrogen production, the characteristic defenses against sexuality are mobilized and become more and more affect-laden as the production of hormones increases. In infantile persons, anxiety and/or hostility toward men may cover up the heterosexual tendencies.

level of psychosexual maturation is not achieved, the woman's regressive wish to be the child herself and to be taken care of is expressed, accompanied usually by a depressive mood.

If impregnation does not occur, the production of progestins declines and the ensuing low hormone level characterizes the premenstrual phase of the cycle. The woman's emotional reactions reveal her perception of "the moderate degree of ovarian deficiency"[1] which the premenstrual phase represents. Parallel with this, a partial regression of the psychosexual integration takes place and *pregenital*—usually anal-sadistic and eliminative—tendencies appear in the motivation of the psychoanalytic material. This, together with the increased general irritability of the sympathetic nervous system, may account for the fact that the premenstrual phase is often described as the *recurrent neurosis of women* (Chadwick—46). Its symptoms show great variations: general apprehension and the fear of bleeding seem to revive the idea that menstruation is identical with castration; thus infantile sexual concepts may return in anxiety dreams and may also motivate irascibility when awake. In other cases, fatigue, crankiness, and weeping spells indicate a depressive condition. The hormonal state itself shows variations, and thus the premenstrual phase has different emotional concomitants in different individuals; it may also change in the same woman from cycle to cycle. The psychoanalytic material of the late premenstrual phase reveals correlations with (a) low hormone level, which is the result of simultaneous decrease in both hormones; (b) declining progestin and incipient estrogen production; and (c) declining progestin and increasing estrogen production. The latter is a constellation in which the eliminative tendency, concurrent with declining progestin, fuses with the heterosexual tendency. The corresponding

[1] R. G. Hoskins: *Endocrinology*. New York, W. W. Norton & Company, Inc., 1941.

emotional state is characterized by an increased tension which lends a "driving" quality to all activities during these days. In many instances, the woman is satisfied that she is doing more work than other times; but most often they complain about the restlessness which accompanies their overactivity. At the same time, the sexual desire shows an urgency which the same woman may not experience in other phases of her sexual cycle. Describing the same phenomena from the point of view of the ego, one may also define it as a regression, as if the ego had been deprived of some of its integrative capacity and is unable to mediate between the various needs; all desires appear imperative, all frustrations unbearable; all emotions are less controlled and the woman appears less composed than during other phases of the sexual cycle. Fortunately, the reaction to the premenstrual hormonal fluctuation does not remain the same during the whole reproductive period of a woman. With further sexual maturation, especially after childbearing, the regressions appear to be absorbed by the adaptive processes of the development.

The end of the sexual cycle is marked by the menstrual flow, which, ushered in by a sudden decrease of hormone production, continues for several days. Soon after the flow is established, the tense mood relaxes, the excitability decreases, and the adult woman accepts menstruation usually with relief. The depressive attitudes are apt to continue from the premenstrual phase into the period of flow. Although this may be explained on a hormonal basis, it is interesting to note that the corresponding psychological material can be interpreted as *regret* over the failure of pregnancy. Women then often recall sad experiences or have remorse about previous abortions; they depreciate the female genitals, which appear to them superfluous; they identify menstrual flow with feces, and thus the genitals are considered dirty and the personality depreciated. After a few days, normally still during the flow, the follicular function of the new cycle begins again and concomitantly sexual stimulation and a state of well-being arises.

This is, indeed, a schematic outline of the sexual cycle, but it may suffice to demonstrate that the cyclic fluctuation of hormones forces the emotional processes of the adult woman into certain regulated channels.

On the other side of the ledger is the influence of emotional factors upon the gonads. The comparative study of a series of cycles of the same woman reveals the effects which stimulating and inhibiting emotional factors have upon the *course* of the gonadal cycle. It is well known that emotions may precipitate or delay the menstrual flow; less known is the fact that the time of ovulation also may vary under similar influences. For example, gratifying or exciting heterosexual intercourse may facilitate ovulation, while frustration or fear may inhibit it. The oscillation in the time of ovulation is such that probably no invariable period of infertility exists in the human species (although this condition is approximately reached in the last week preceding menstruation). In the same way, the number of ovulations, the frequency of anovulatory cycles, and the symptoms of the premenstrual phase— more in some women and less in others—are also influenced by emotional factors. The comparative study of the sexual cycles of several individuals reveals that the pattern of the cycle unfolds in accordance with the constitutional and environmental factors which determine the structure of the personality. The most obvious characteristic of the cycle is its length—i.e., the interval between two menstruations. The average length is 28 days; some women menstruate in 21- to 23-day intervals; others, also within the range of normal, have cycles of 32 to 35 days' duration. Most revealing for the pattern of the hormonal cycle is the intricate relationship between the estrogen and progestin phases of the cycle.

Progestin is the specifically female hormone. While estrogen may be produced in varying degrees from childhood on (and in both sexes), progestin develops only after puberty as a function of the ovum. It is understandable that its relation to estrogen production, its relative deficiency or its preponderance, determines the variations of the cycle. If the individual reaches normal sexual maturity without fixating traumata in the pregenital phases, the hormone cycles—i.e., the relationship between the estrogen and progestin phases of the cycle—will be normal; this implies practically normal ovulation and normal length of the cycle. If—either because of constitution or crippling traumata, or on account of the interaction of both—fixation occurs on a pregenital level, the disturbance of the psychosexual maturation will be reflected in the cycle. For example, in puerile, bisexual individuals, the progestin phase does not develop fully; they usually have short cycles. Women whose infantile fixation causes a prevalence of receptive-retentive tendencies (for example, cases of bulimia, obesity) usually have long progesterone phases and also long cycles. If the psychosexual development is even more inhibited, long low-hormone periods characterize the cycle; menstrual flow may occur with irregularities within the normal range. While the pattern of the hormonal cycle unfolds concomitantly with those factors which determine the psychosexual development, the psychodynamic course of the cycle seems to repeat the development in condensed form again and again under the stimulus of the hormonal cycle.

The study of the sexual cycle permits significant conclusions in regard to the organization of the female sexual drive. Corresponding to the two phases of the female sexual function, it has two tendencies which act consecutively: an *active* tendency, the aim of which is to secure the sexual act, and a *passive* (receptive-retentive) tendency, which acts to secure the functions of pregnancy. Helene Deutsch (63), through psychoanalytic observations, came to the conclusion that a "tendency toward introversion" and a "deep-rooted passivity" are the specific qualities of the female psyche. The study of the sexual cycle confirms this view and determines its physiological substratum. Since these tendencies become manifest at periodic intervals, parallel with the activity of the specifically female gonad hormone, progestin, we are justified in assuming that the psychodynamic tendencies which prepare emotionally for motherhood represent a genuine quality of the female psychosexual anlage.

PREGNANCY

When pregnancy occurs, the cyclic function of the ovaries is interrupted and is not re-established with regularity until after lactation is finished. The psychology of pregnancy—its basic psychodynamic processes—is readily understood in the light of what is known about the psychology of the progestin phase. The receptive and retentive tendencies and the tendency for introversion of psychic energies characterize pregnancy also; the intensity, however, is multiplied manyfold, corresponding with the highly increased hormone production.

The interaction between mother and fetus—the symbiosis —begins after conception (Benedek—26). The enhanced hormonal and general metabolic processes which are necessary to maintain pregnancy again produce "surplus energy" and replenish the reservoir of the mother's primary narcissism. The pregnant woman in her vegetative calmness enjoys her body, which is abundant with libidinous feelings. This enhances her well-being and becomes the source of her motherliness. The primary narcissistic gratification of pregnancy increases the mother's patience in regard to the discomforts of pregnancy. Another factor in the psychology of pregnancy is expressed by the intensification of the receptive tendencies. This is the manifestation of the biological process of growth which it serves. Not only may the pregnant woman want to "eat for two"; [1] her dependent needs are also revived. She thrives on the solicitude of her environment, and if her dependent wishes are unfulfilled, the resulting sense of frustration increases the tension of her receptive needs, which may destroy the primary narcissistic state of pregnancy and thus interfere with the development of motherliness.

Though pregnancy is biologically normal, it is an exceptional condition, which tests the physical and psychological reserves of the woman. While her total metabolic and emotional economy is concentrated upon the tasks of pregnancy, her ego appears regressed if measured by the usual level of its integration. At the same time, on a biological level, the span of the total personality expands to encompass her child. If the mother feels her growing capacity to love and to take care of the child, then she experiences a general improvement of her emotional state. Many neurotic women who at other times suffer from anxiety become free from it during pregnancy; others become free from depressions and from desperate mood changes. Many women, despite physical discomfort and nausea, feel emotionally stable and have a "good time" during pregnancy. Whether the general metabolic and hormonal stimulation is primarily responsible for such improvement, or whether gratification because the personality achieves its goal in procreation can account for it, remains to be evaluated clinically and probably varies from case to case.

PARTURITION

Recent studies by Dunbar (219) and others have attempted to evaluate the influence which the mother's psychological attitude has upon the process of parturition. They have employed various methods of "mental hygiene" during the supervision of pregnancy to diminish the woman's fear of the

[1] Dr. Thomas S. Szasz in two recent papers (224, 225) discusses the hypersalivation occurring during pregnancy in the light of the regressive phenomena of the autonomic nervous system.

delivery. On the other hand, modern obstetrics employs hypnosis and various forms of anesthesia to render parturition painless. How much these procedures help the mother to recover from the delivery with the happy feelings of motherliness, and in what respect these procedures interfere with it, have to be evaluated on extensive case material. No doubt there are many instances in which the obstetrical trauma has alienated the mother from her child. But the great majority of women have delivered and still deliver their babies without anesthesia; they usually recover quickly and smile happily at the child. It is common knowledge that women soon forget the pains of birth. There are also many modern women who, having delivered the baby under anesthesia, feel deprived of the great sensation of motherhood; they complain that the lack of memory of the delivery made it difficult for them to accept the baby as their own and to feel "motherly" toward him.

Parturition interrupts the biological symbiosis between mother and infant. The process is traumatic not only for the infant, but for the mother also. The hormonal changes which induce and control parturition, the labor pains and the excitement, even without the use of narcotics, interrupt the emotional continuity of the mother-child unity. During delivery, the mother is concentrated upon her survival. After delivery, the love for the new-born wells up in her as she first hears the cry of the baby. With the feeling of a "good job well done," she relaxes; her organism prepares for the next function of motherhood—*lactation*.

Lactation is a function which is stimulated and maintained by a specific hormone of the anterior lobe of the pituitary gland, *prolactin*. The influence of prolactin upon the performance of the tasks of motherliness is well studied in animals. In the human, one is inclined to neglect the purely physiological aspects of such a highly valued achievement as motherliness. The physiological preparation for lactation indicates that the mother's body after parturition is not yet ready to give up the symbiosis with her infant: lactation represents an extrauterine (partial) symbiosis between mother and child. The psychodynamic concomitants of lactation are similar to those of the progestin phase of the cycle.[1] During this phase, the intention toward motherliness is expressed by active and passive receptive tendencies. During lactation, these tendencies gain in intensity; they become the axis around which the activities of motherliness center. The mother's desire to nurse the baby, to be close to it bodily, represents the continuation of the original symbiosis, and this produces pleasurable tactile sensations, not only in the infant, but also in the mother. While the infant incorporates the breast, the mother feels united with her baby. The identification with the baby permits the mother to "regress"—i.e., to repeat and satisfy her own passive-receptive, dependent needs. Through the process of identification between mother and child, lactation permits a slow, step-by-step integration of normal motherliness. If this process of the mother's development is suppressed, the enforced changes in the hormonal function may disturb the psychosomatic balance which is the source of motherliness.

The vulnerability of the woman's development to motherliness can be explained by a summary of the psychosomatic processes of the puerperium and lactation: this phase in the mother's life is dominated by *oral-receptive tendencies*. That the intensification of the oral-receptive tendencies represents the psychodynamic conditions for the development of depression is a well-established concept of psychoanalysis. (Abraham, Freud—3, 93). Thus the psychodynamic tendencies con-

[1] Prolactin and estrogen act as antagonists. During pregnancy, the high estrogen production suppresses mammary function; during normal lactation, prolactin inhibits the estrogen production. Most women, therefore, do not ovulate or menstruate during lactation.

comitant with motherhood and nursing predispose the woman to self-criticism in regard to the same functions. She becomes oversensitive in regard to her ability to be a good mother. Every indication of her failure—the crying of the baby, for example—increases her sense of inferiority and may create anxious tension and depression in her. As the suppression of lactation may interfere with motherliness, so failure of motherliness, originating in other sources of the personality, may interfere with lactation. Folk knowledge had always assumed that the mother's emotional state influenced her capacity to nurse the baby; if she were happy, her milk was "good" and the baby thrived on it; if she were unhappy, depressed, or excited, the quantity and quality of her milk changed and caused colic and other suffering in the baby. It is the task of further study of the external symbiosis between mother and child to provide a scientific explanation for these challenging observations.

When lactation is finished, the mother's reproductive task with one child is completed; the cyclic function of the ovaries is re-established in order to prepare her for the next offspring. Through the cyclic repetition of the preparation for motherhood and through the fulfillment of this instinctual need, the woman reaches her sexual maturation as well as the completion of the development of her personality.

THE MENOPAUSE

The reproductive period in women lasts, on the average, about thirty-five years. Its decline approaches gradually; its end is marked by the cessation of the menstrual flow—*menopause*—which occurs during the period of "change of life"—i.e., during the climacteric or climacterium. In our culture, this period is usually anticipated with apprehension, since women assume that the climacterium represents a period of severe mental and physical stress. Yet there are many women who hardly notice the transition; others suffer, for a longer or shorter period, from restlessness and irritability, from insomnia, palpitation, and "hot flashes"—i.e., from symptoms which can be attributed to the instability of the autonomic nervous system. There is evidence of a difference in the process of tissue degeneration of the ovaries in women who have not borne children as against those who have had several pregnancies. The menopause sets in earlier and with more intense reactions in the former group than in the latter. This finding is in harmony with psychoanalytic observations—namely, that with complete sexual maturation and function, the regressive emotional manifestations, which characterize the low ebb of the premenstrual hormone phase, become absorbed by the adaptive processes of development. Thus when the gonadal stimulation subsides permanently, the emotional economy of the healthy woman is not severely threatened by this loss. With the integration of the personality once established, the woman becomes independent of gonadal stimulation for maintaining the sublimations achieved during the reproductive period.

Women who were unable to adapt to the monthly premenstrual hormone decline and had premenstrual depressions and dysmenorrhea are apt to suffer again from the discomforts of the climacterium. Many women suffer from neurotic, somatic, and even psychotic manifestations which, because they occur about the time of the menopause, are often attributed to the stresses of the climacterium. But the psychoanalytic study of such cases reveals that the symptoms which appear aggravated during climacterium had already existed (or if latent, had been preformed) in the precarious balance of the personality during the reproductive period. The life history and the personality structure in a great percentage of these cases reveal that (1) the bisexual disposition played a disturbing role in the development and (2) the psychic economy was

dominated—much like that of men's—by strivings of the ego
rather than by the primary emotional gratifications of motherliness.[1]

The climacterium is different in those women whose adaptive capacity has not been exhausted by previous neurotic
processes. When the cessation of biological growth releases
psychic energy which was previously employed in the reproductive tasks, this gives the flexible ego of such women new
impetus for learning and socialization. The manifold interests and productivities of women after the climacterium, as
well as the improvement in their general physical and emotional health, prompts us to regard the climacterium, in the
psychological sense, as a developmental phase (Benedek—25).

3. PSYCHOSEXUAL DYSFUNCTIONS

The dysfunctions of sexuality are often distinguished as
manifestations of *hypo-* and *hyper*-sexuality. The foregoing
discussion indicates, however, that such distinction has
descriptive rather than psychodynamic or endocrinological significance. The terms designating the various symptoms of
sexual dysfunctions do not refer to well-defined nosological
entities. The symptoms may change in the same individual
from one to another, motivated not only by more or less
permanent developmental changes in psychodynamics, but also
by transitory circumstances which influence the mood and increase or decrease the desire, as well as the anxiety related to
sexual intercourse.

Sexual inhibition may be felt as shyness toward the opposite sex, or as lack of interest in, or antipathy toward, sexual
activity. It may be rationalized by fear of venereal disease,
as well as by the cultural demands for chastity. These emotions as well as their rationalizations serve as defenses against

---

[1] Expressed in terms of hormones, we may say that the estrogen phase over-
balances the progestin phase in the sexual cycle of these women.

more significant sexual conflicts, which may remain repressed as long as sexual intercourse is avoided. In this sense, impotence in men and frigidity in women can be considered as defenses of the ego.

Impotence is a symptom which deeply offends the man's self-esteem. It serves as protection against conflicts and impulses which might become threatening to the self if the ego controls were lessened by sexual ecstasy. Impotence, for example, may keep in repression sadistic impulses and fantasies. The fantasy that the penis is a powerful destructive organ which could do irrevocable harm to the loved woman is but the denial and projection of the *castration anxiety, which is the basic motivation of all sexual inhibitions*. The fear of losing the penis may interfere with developing erections, or it may cause loss of erection ante portas. The severity of impotence may be measured by the strength or weakness of the erections. In light cases, impotence may be the result of a "negative conditioning," so to speak. After the man has experienced failure, shame and apprehension may counteract his erection when intercourse is next attempted. Impotence represents a more severe symptom if motivated by conflicting bisexual tendencies; in such cases, erection may subside quickly, or may not develop completely. The psychodynamic motivation of impotence is then closely related to that of *ejaculatio praecox*.

Ejaculatio praecox may vary in intensity and in frequency. The light cases are characterized by the shortness of the act and/or by the tendency for a passive outflow of the seminal fluid without the muscular rhythm of orgasm. This may occasionally occur in men of normal potency. It may happen, namely, that the eliminative urge, which is one element of the orgastic act, overpowers the other, the withholding, retaining element. Such an incident may occur after long abstinence. Then the pressure of the seminal fluid seems to enforce a quick discharge, illustrating the fact that the male sexual organs have a primarily eliminative function. Abraham (1) studied the various forms of ejaculatio praecox and described their dynamics, to which little has since been added. Ejaculatio praecox represents a fixation on *urethral eroticism*. This libidinal fixation is usually "trained" by enuresis and masturbation and is therefore connected with guilt and with inferiority feelings; it usually leads to an unconscious identification of semen with urine, which brings about the impulse to eliminate immediately when pressure is felt.[1] This indicates that those who suffer from ejaculatio praecox have not integrated with the primary passive-eliminative tendency the active, aggressive-eliminative component of the sexual drive without which the genital primacy of the penis cannot be achieved. Only a rhythmic change between such active eliminative and retentive tendencies creates orgasm. Abraham recognized the feminine orientation of the leading erotogenic zone in the case of ejaculatio praecox: the climax of excitement is felt at the root of the penis and on the perineum rather than at the glans and in the shaft of the penis. This indicates that ejaculatio praecox is motivated by the feminine component of the sexual anlage which, in the process of sexual maturation, has not been mastered and superseded.

Ejaculatio retardata is symptomatically the opposite of ejaculatio praecox: the tendency to retain overpowers the tendency to eliminate and thus interferes with orgastic discharge. This symptom may also occur in individuals of normal potency, especially after sexual exhaustion. As a pathological symptom, it expresses the anxiety connected with the loss of semen. While the castration anxiety, in these cases, does not affect the desire for and the power of erection and intromission, the ejaculation is inhibited by the anxiety of losing the self, or by the fear of death. Therefore, the retaining, originally anal-sadistic tendency takes over the regulation of the orgastic rhythm. It

---

1 This does not explain why there is such a resistance against retaining urine and controlling the sphincter. The symptom represents regression to an early phase of infantile functioning when the bladder was passively emptied, without the necessity of overcoming the tension of the sphincter.

would not be surprising if closer observation would reveal that the symptom is related to functional sterility in men.

The fact that urethral eroticism is closely interwoven with infantile genital eroticism is responsible for the symptom of *enuresis*. This condition usually occurs during the latency period, and in the great majority of cases it is overcome when the gonad function sets in. The disappearance of enuresis at puberty is probably the result of the maturation of the sexual organs. The excitation which used to be discharged by the pregenital urinary eroticism becomes displaced to the genital organs and is discharged by nocturnal emissions.[1] However, there are cases in which enuresis persists after puberty.

The preoccupation with urinary eroticism in childhood leaves traces in the psychosexual household which may be reawakened by other than sexual stimulation. Not only libidinal gratifications provoke the child's preoccupation with urination; the first ego gratifications and the sense of mastery are also connected with the learning of sphincter control. Thus much of the child's self-esteem develops in connection with his first much-praised achievement. Later, during the latency period, the ego's striving for mastery, its ambition for success in competition, is expressed and remains forever connected with urethral eroticism (Jones—127). Therefore, excitations originally not sexual in nature become discharged by the urinary tract. For example, anxious tension, especially if the anxiety is related to ego performance and achievement, may cause *increased diuresis*. The kidneys fill the bladder with large quantities of urine (of very low specific gravity) and compel a preoccupation with bladder control and urination. Some individuals erotize the process to such a degree that the drinking of large quantities of water and the ensuing dis-

---

[1] In girls, the equivalent of nocturnal emission, orgasm, can hardly be responsible for the cessation of enuresis after puberty. With the maturation of the sexual organs, other tendencies gain intensity and take over the discharge of sexual excitation.

charge of large quantities of urine imitates diabetes insipidus. In other cases, the polyuria itself activates anxiety in regard to bladder control; the fear of "being late" activates a sado-masochistic tension and *urinary frequency.* This enforced urination may be accompanied by *spermatorrhea.* This is a leakage in which seminal fluid (or mostly prostatic secretions) escapes. Masturbation, or rather the fear of its results, may cause this symptom in younger men; however, it occurs more commonly in older men, especially in the presence of an enlarged prostate and preoccupations with urinary frequency. It may then be one of the symptoms of the *male climacteric.*

The term *climacteric,* or *climacterium,* is often applied to the period of abating reproductive function in both sexes. The process differs in the male and female according to the different organizations of the reproductive function. There is no definite cessation of the reproductive period in men comparable to the menopause in women. In men, not only the sexual urge, but also the reproductive capacity may be rekindled, even after they appear to be already extinguished. Nevertheless, with the advancing years, the sexual capacity declines noticeably. The way in which the individual responds to his waning sexual potency depends upon the total organization of the personality. The well-balanced individual takes it in his stride, finding compensations in his achievements and in his family. Some individuals, however—especially those of marked narcissistic character formation—may respond to insecurity about potency with a regression. Since a failure in potency may appear as an irreparable damage to the personality, it may activate the ever-latent castration fear; this, in turn, motivates the symptoms which make the assumption of a *male climacterium* justifiable. In some cases, with the loss of vigor, the erotization of regressive tendencies may occur; then urinary disorders, as described above, may develop. In other instances, the effort to keep up the potency, when the integrating effect of androgens is already dissipated, reawakens infantile fantasies and tendencies toward sexual perversion. A pseudo hypersexuality may thus develop. Since the involutional period is one in which the gonadal hormone is known to be deficient, the perversions which may accompany it indicate that perversions do not represent hypersexuality in a physiological sense. They represent fixations on and regressions to pregenital sexual tendencies (Fenichel—83).

The term *homosexuality*, loosely used, includes all sexual practices between members of the same sex. The psychodynamic motivations of each variety of homosexual perversion are well established, beginning with the simple arresting of heterosexual development and including those of functional intergrade sexual conditions in which erotic feeling for the opposite sex appears inconceivable. However, correlations of psychodynamic constellations, with bodily and hormonal indicators of the sexual aberrations, are lacking. In some cases of homosexuality—but not in all of them and not in simple relation to the severity of the perversion—some aspects of the build of the body, the hair growth, gait, and gestures reveal that homosexuality is deeply ingrained, not only in the emotional, but also in the physical make-up. There have been several attempts to solve the riddle by determining the supposed endocrine imbalance, for the purpose of proving that a reversed androgen-estrogen ratio is the basis of homosexuality. Since the variations of this indicator of bisexuality are great in so-called normal individuals as well, the results do not solve the problem of homosexuality. There are cases in the literature in which implantation of testicular grafts changed the direction of the libido. Hormone therapy usually fails, however, since the increased hormonal tension requires discharge in a homosexual direction (Perloff—179). In spite of this, psychoanalytic therapy seems to achieve a change in the psychodynamic constellations only in those cases in which the developmental retardation outweighs the biological motivating factors.

Hypersexuality and/or precocious maturity is described in the literature; there are no psychoanalytic studies of such individuals. There are some indications that the pregenital tendencies, which reach such preponderance in the psychosexual household as to give rise to lasting perversions, might have represented a partial precociousness, a partial hypersexuality in childhood. To express this in psychodynamic terms: partial instinctual tendencies may absorb such a great part of the available libido that, as a result, they cannot be integrated in the developmental process of sexuality; isolated, they drive toward independent discharge. Such partial discharge cannot channelize all sexual energy completely. Thus the need for gratification of the partial tendencies arises in quick sequences; they appear insatiable. Therefore, perversions give the impression of hypersexuality. But measured on the total psychosexual balance, the minus quantity will be evident in the diminished orgastic potency.

All the manifestations of hypo- and hypersexuality discussed here—except that of the male climacterium—demonstrate that the dysfunctions of the sexual apparatus are motivated by intrapsychic conflicts and thus by the internal consumption of psychosexual energy; somatic as their symptoms may be, they have no endocrinological correlate massive enough to be detected by the present methods of endocrinology. They are, in the real sense of the word, *psychosexual dysfunctions*.

The psychosexual dysfunctions of women are easily related to the function of the ovaries, since this is expressed quite directly in variations of the sexual cycle and in variations of the menstrual symptoms.

Frigidity, the most frequent psychosexual dysfunction, can, however, be related to the ovarian function only in rare cases of severe hypogonadism. In all other instances, women may have any form and degree of frigidity and, at the same time, normal gonadal function. No doubt many women have children and become good mothers without ever having experienced orgasm. For, in women more so than in men, the quality of the sexual experience depends upon the mate, upon his potency and skill, upon his ability to overcome her shyness and her sexual fear. There are, of course, women whose orgastic capacity is uninhibited and who also, by the anatomical constitution of the sexual apparatus, achieve orgasm easily. The complexity of sexual maturation in women, with all its cultural complications, is apt to create defenses against sexuality which are expressed by inhibitions of the woman's capacity for orgasm. The psychodynamic motivations of frigidity are the same as those of impotence. Frigidity is rooted in anxiety about the danger which remains unconsciously associated with the attainment of the sexual aim: in women, the fear of being damaged by the penis and the fear of pregnancy and childbirth. Yet the social and emotional significance of frigidity is very different from that of impotence. Frigidity is no obstacle to the reproductive function, as is impotence. Since female orgasm should be achieved by "passive co-operation," its failure does not offend the woman's self-esteem as much as impotence hurts the man's. Sexual practices which may help to overcome the woman's frigidity may often represent an obstacle in the man's own gratification; hence frigidity is often regarded as of negligible significance. In some mores—like those of the Victorian era in Western culture—orgasm was regarded as "unwomanly," and not having orgasm was considered to be a virtue. It is well established that conversion hysteria is a correlate of the repression of sexuality required by such mores. Today frigidity is not considered a virtue, but a lack, for which women sometimes blame themselves and more often their husbands. While women admit their reactions to the frustration of their need for orgasm, their response depends upon the structure of the total personality.

There are women who, in a sort of "motherly giving" attitude, are satisfied by partial gratification; others respond with anger and depression; still others, being afraid of frustration, anxiously watch the sexual act and control it with hostility; they thus interfere with what they want to achieve, as far as their conscious self knows. The emotional manifestations reveal the underlying sexual conflict, usually based upon the conflicting bisexual tendencies which impede the orgastic capacity.

Vaginismus is the extreme manifestation of the bisexual conflict and of the resulting sexual fear. This symptom represents the displacement of the expected sexual excitation to the perineal and vaginal muscles. While it protects the woman from the pain of which she is afraid, she suffers a self-created pain. Omitting here the sexual fantasies which this symptom expresses, vaginismus achieves its goal by excluding the penis, by expelling it, or by painfully enclosing it. No doubt, sadistic and masochistic tendencies fuse in this symptom with urethral and anal eliminative and retentive tendencies. Thus, the symptom can be paralleled with ejaculatio praecox and/or with ejaculatio retardata. Since the vagina is a receptive organ, vaginismus is an expression of powerful oral-incorporative tendencies; it seems to be the realization of the threatening idea of the "vagina dentata." Vaginismus occurs usually in young women whose psychosexual make-up reveals, besides the urethral and anal fixation, also their sexual infantilism. This is expressed not only in their emotional life, but also in the incompleteness and immaturity of their sexual cycles. Yet the physiological and psychological aspects of the phenomena cannot be considered independently. If the sexual cycle of the woman who responds to her sexual frustration with anger and depression shows, parallel with this mood, declining ovarian hormone production, it cannot be determined with our present methods of investigation whether the low hormone level causes the dissatisfied mood or whether the anger and frustration suppress the hormone production. Women with more labile hormonal function seem apt to be frigid. It is, however, justifiable to ask whether the interaction of the factors which cause frigidity may also influence the ovarian functions through the medium of frustration and anger. It is well to keep in mind that the sexual cycle, once established, does not represent a stable, unchangeable pattern; this also gives a clue to the complexities of dysmenorrhea.

Dysmenorrhea (Dunbar—75) refers to the physical and emotional disorders which may occur twenty-four to seventy-two hours before, or soon after, the onset of the menstrual flow. In the pathogenesis of this syndrome, two aspects have always been recognized: (1) the physical, which was thought to be a lack of complete sexual maturity, and (2) the emotional, which was designated by the term "psychogenic factors." Symptoms of dysmenorrhea vary greatly, although the same individual usually has essentially the same symptom group with each dysmenorrheal state. Some women suffer from pains resembling those of labor and discharge blood clots; others suffer from hyperemia and distention of the pelvic organs; still others have "membraneous dysmenorrhea" and discharge the hyperplastic mucosa with much pain. No wonder that these women—usually girls—dread the menstruation and prepare for it as for an expected operation. The most frequent form of dysmenorrhea is "menstrual colic": abdominal distress, nausea, vomiting, diarrhea are its usual symptoms; migraine and other vasomotor symptoms, tachycardia or bradycardia, anxiety states, and fainting spells may develop with any of these conditions. The emotional manifestations of the premenstrual tension and depression may develop without any of the physical symptoms of dysmenorrhea. However, they may appear with "menstrual colic" and accompany it with a sort of helpless wrath. The symptoms of premenstrual tension may imitate an agitated depression: a sense of frustration, anger, and restlessness fills the unhappy, unloving mood. The other type of premenstrual depression is characterized by increased sensitivity, sadness, and hypochondriacal anxiety. (These depresions are sufficiently severe so that, as long as they last, women lose sight of the fact that the condition lasts for a few days only.)

Generally, the symptoms of dysmenorrhea and premenstrual depression have the same psychodynamic motivation as the symptoms which represent the normal concomitants of the late premenstrual phase; in dysmenorrhea, however, the symptom manifestations are highly exaggerated. For example, the emotional manifestations which correspond to declining progesterone are motivated by the anal eliminative and retentive tendencies. In normal cases, these tendencies are expressed in dreams and in emotional reactions to the menstruation (it is dirty, etc.), while in the case of dysmenorrhea, the same tendencies motivate the autonomic discharge of the "menstrual colic." This in itself represents a complex and interesting problem. According to psychoanalytic concepts, this general nervous excitation could be explained by the anxiety which menstruation originally mobilized in these individuals, to which is added the fear of a repetition of the suffering. Physiologically, it is known that ovarian deficiency increases the irritability of the autonomic nervous system. But dysmenorrhea does not occur in correspondence with low hormone production only; it is often a concomitant of high estrogen production in the late premenstrual phase and during the menstrual flow.

The following clinical facts may help to clarify this problem: (1) Dysmenorrhea rarely occurs in puberty; it usually develops in the later phases of adolescence. (2) It may occur in women who have had completely normal menstruation and have had children; but, after maturity, a regression may activate dysmenorrhea. An example of the first type of case:

> This was a young woman who began to menstruate when she was 13; she had no "troubles"; her flow was not profuse and

came irregularly in six-to-eight-week intervals. When she was eighteen and in college, she had several more or less serious flirtations; with these, she developed extremely severe dysmenorrhea, for which she was treated for two and a half years with hormone injections. Her menstruation became more regular in time, but the dysmenorrhea remained just as severe; after she married, her dysmenorrhea became complicated by severe premenstrual tension. During her psychoanalysis, vaginal smears revealed a deficient cycle; she had normal estrogen phases and deficient progesterone phases. (She was sterile.) This suggests that the dysmenorrhea began when the erotic stimulation made sexuality an emotional demand, and at the same time it activated her resistance, her rebellion against the "feminine role." Her hormonal cycle revealed that, according to the level of her psychosexual maturation, she had an overbalance of estrogen stimulation, which may account for the dysmenorrhea.

An example of the second variety of cases.

A young married woman had no menstrual difficulties before marriage. She became pregnant easily, and she had two children (age difference between them—two and a half years). When her second child was about a year and a half old, she suddenly felt strong aggressive impulses toward her children. She became panicky; she fought her panic with phobic reactions. Along with this, she developed severe dysmenorrhea. Her feeling about menstruation was that it equates abortion and that she suffered because she did not want more children. Her emotional cycle had shown the fight against motherhood. Thus we assume that, corresponding and in response to her severe anxiety state, a regression took place. In this case, we assume that the anxiety and guilty feelings increased the tonus of the autonomic nervous system and, at the same time, disturbed the balance of the hormonal cycle; the two factors together are responsible for the dysmenorrhea.

The psychodynamic responses to the late premenstrual phase are usually more intense and more complex than could be expected on the basis of the ovarian hormone production alone. In cases of dysmenorrhea, the specificity of the psychodynamic reactions are overshadowed by the autonomic nervous system reaction. Dysmenorrhea, although it represents a reaction to deficient (infantile type) ovarian function, is not a symptom of hyposexuality alone. It is rather a result of the diminishing control of the ego over the psychosexual conflicts. The conflicts, "returning from repression," mobilize anxiety and general nervous system reactions, which, in turn, predispose the woman to an overreaction to the premenstrual hormonal change.

Oligomenorrhea means scanty menstruation at long intervals. It may be the sign of retarded sexual maturation on the basis of hypogonadism, but more often it occurs secondarily, as a result of psychic regression. This was found, for example, in cases of bulimia and the ensuing alimentary obesity. Bulimia may develop in women who respond to the female sexual function, not with masculine identification, but with depression and with regression to the oral phase of development. The metabolic processes of obesity as well as the depression may be responsible for the manifestations of hyposexuality, which usually respond well to psychotherapy.

Amenorrhea is a more serious form of oligomenorrhea. The two manifestations may interchange. Amenorrhea may be a sign of hypogonadism, but it may also occur as a result of psychogenic influences. Among the psychogenic cases of amenorrhea, two main groups may be differentiated. One is the amenorrhea of young women who, in their defense against feminine sexuality, are able to repress the ovarian cycle more or less completely; with it, usually, the emotional manifestations of sexuality are not repressed. Thus they may go on fantasying about a life rich in heterosexual experiences without having anything to do with the "dirty, painful, disagreeable" part of femininity. No doubt, an organic disposition facilitates such an outcome; for similar intensity of psychosexual conflict and even greater intensity of anxiety in other cases motivate other symptoms, less interfering with the reproductive function. However, these cases respond well to analytic psychotherapy. After they become able to experience hetero-sexual stimulation, the amenorrhea usually disappears.

The other form of amenorrhea occurs as a part of the syn-drome of *pseudocyesis* or "grossesse nerveuse." These terms refer to cases of amenorrhea in which the woman firmly be-lieves that she is pregnant and develops objective pregnancy signs, in the absence of pregnancy. It occurs quite often that, under the influence of the wish for and the fear of pregnancy, the early symptoms of pregnancy appear, delaying menstrua-tion for many weeks. The much-reported cases of amenorrhea of long duration with abdominal distention and with breast changes, imitating pregnancy, are complex psychosexual, usually conversion-hysterical symptoms. The symptom ex-presses the conflicts regarding childbearing on several levels. Usually these women are sterile. Being unconsciously afraid of pregnancy and guilty because of the often conscious hostil-ity toward children, these women consciously clamor for motherhood and, during the period of pseudocyesis, enjoy the gratification which only pregnancy justifies.

The psychopathological manifestations of the reproductive functions are manifold. The reproductive urge—being but a special manifestation of the instinct of self-preservation—may be in conflict in each step with the interests, wishes, and de-sires of the self. This plays a role in the sexual pathology of men, too. In women, the conflict between self-preservation and the propagative function appears warranted, since child-bearing may be dangerous and the tasks of motherhood are burdensome. What has been said about the instinctual tend-encies for motherhood, its developmental integration during sexual maturation, and its manifestations during each sexual cycle, exposes also the conflicts which may lead to various pathological manifestations of the reproductive function. Women are usually unaware of their conflicts regarding child-bearing until the conflicts become activated by the intensive psychic and metabolic processes of pregnancy. The emotional disturbance related to pregnancy may be described as a *hypochondriasis*. Hypochondriasis is the result of the concentration of (narcissistic) libido, which is perceived with anxious and worrisome awareness of the organ or organs which represent a source of danger (Ferenczi—84). Thus the same narcissistic cathexis which accounts for the contentment during normal pregnancy may provoke an intolerable anxiety if the woman's ego senses nothing but danger in motherhood. Analysis of the individual case will reveal whether the anxiety originates in the reactions to the bodily changes of pregnancy, and in the anticipation of the dangers of childbirth, or whether it is primarily caused by hostility toward the yet unborn child. In some cases, anxiety regarding the body causes only hypochondriacal symptoms; in other instances, the mobilized aggression may be projected on the child, who is hated and feared as the cause of all the disturbance. In some instances, the primary aggression toward the child sets in motion a depression which may lead secondarily to hypochondriasis.

Psychoanalytic study of the various disturbances of pregnancy reveals that the same psychodynamic conflicts may be responsible for different pathological phenomena. We may assume that constitutional factors [1] determine whether the developmental conflict will affect the somatic (hormonal and metabolic) processes of pregnancy or whether the same conflict will activate psychiatric disturbances. In some cases, the fear of the pregnancy and/or the hostile impulses toward the child may act through suppression of the hormonal processes which sustain pregnancy, thus causing abortion; in other cases, toxic vomiting or anorexia nervosa develops without any conscious awareness of the emotional conflict. In the "purely" psychiatric cases, the pregnancy may progress normally but the woman is suddenly stricken by panic which is

[1] All other endocrine glands, besides the ovaries, especially the pituitary, the adrenals, and the thyroid, may be involved.

rationalized by ideas of the harm which the growing fetus causes inside the body, or by fear of death in childbirth; the panic may be increased by suicidal impulses or by aggressive impulses toward the child. In the defensive struggle against the panic, the woman may develop phobic reactions or depressions, or may regress to severe schizophrenic psychosis ("post-partum psychosis"). In some cases, interruption of the pregnancy or parturition may lead to symptomatic recovery; in other cases, it does not arrest the process, which, once started, makes the woman feel inferior and guilty because she failed in her natural function. It seems that the onrushing metabolic processes of pregnancy recharge the developmental conflicts with such intense emotions that they overwhelm the ego and render it helpless in the face of the most significant integrative task in a woman's life.

More fortunate, in some respects, are those women who are saved from the realization of their conflicts in regard to childbearing by *sterility*. The study of the various manifestations of the inhibitions of the reproductive functions shows that fertility is relative. Infertility may be absolute in cases of pelvic and glandular abnormalities due to developmental defects and disease. All other forms of infertility are relative, depending upon a great variety of organic (metabolic) and psychic factors. And here we may repeat: so far as the psychodynamic motivations of sterility are known, the same conflicts which cause a hypochondriacal panic in one woman and depression in another may be elicited in connection with sterility in still another. The women who "suffer" from functional sterility are unaware of their anxieties and hostilities in regard to childbearing; they may go on asserting their unambivalent attitude toward motherhood.

So-called "functional sterility" has many variations; in some cases it may not amount to a real psychosomatic symptom because there is no somatic change. For example, a woman may appear sterile when the desire for intercourse is suppressed during the fertile period and coitus takes place only during the infertile phase of the cycle. The somatic change leading to infertility may be a shift in the cycle so that ovulation occurs during menstruation, when coitus usually does not take place (Rubenstein—197, 198). Thus the neurotic change of the desire for parenthood in either or in both marital partners may initiate sterility and as a result of the interaction between the marital partners, it may lead finally to suppression of fertility. There is greater organic compliance in the cases where sterility is caused by spasm of the Fallopian tubes and their closure, and also in those cases where the psychosexual conflicts lead to a suppresion of the ovarian function so that ovulation does not occur.

The motivations of functional sterility can best be studied by analyzing the woman's reaction to her infertility. The psychology of adoption, intriguing as it may be, cannot be included here. Yet the motivations which urge the woman to adopt a child after she knows of her sterility afford insight into the psychology of motherhood as well as of sterility. Some women, urged by their natural motherliness, are eager to expend this on a child; if it cannot be their own, the adopted child is emotionally accepted as a substitute.[1] In other women, the urge for adoption covers the sense of inferiority, the damage to the ego caused by sterility; for some others, the adoption appears as a welcome solution for all problems, since, besides other satisfactions, it relieves the mother (the father as well, for that matter) from the anxieties and from the narcissistic conflicts which one may have in regard to the endowments of one's own child. All these factors indicate the complex involvement of the ego in parenthood. That such influences suffice to suppress the woman's ability to bear children is demonstrated by the cases in which the woman becomes fer-

[1] This occurs mostly in situations in which a not sterile, motherly woman accepts the sterility of her husband and is able to become a good mother for the adopted child.

tile after she adopts a child. Although there are only few such cases published (Orr—176), this is not a rare occurrence. It seems that after the woman has been able to accept a child and "practice" her motherliness, her anxiety diminishes sufficiently to make conception possible.

It remains to speculate about the causes of the different degrees of susceptibility of the reproductive apparatus to the influence of the emotions. Since the conflicts motivated by the environment are limited and the responses to them differ in high degree, we may ask what are the constitutional factors which account for the intensification of the conflict on the psychological side. As a broad generalization, we may refer to bisexuality. On the organic side, constitutional factors may account for that vulnerability of the endocrine system which permits sterility.

The total or partial deficiency of gonadotropin causes failure of the gonads. *Hypogonadism* may occur in both sexes; the significance of its effect upon the personality, in both sexes, depends upon the cause and degree of hypogonadism and upon the age when the deficiency became effective. In men, deficiency of gonadotropin causes *eunuchoidism. Cryptorchidism* (the failure of the testes to descend into the scrotum) is also the result of the deficiency of gonadotropin and may lead to varying degrees of eunuchoidism. Castration, by accident, by surgery, or by disease such as mumps or tuberculosis, also causes hypogonadism. Male eunuchoidism is more conspicuous, probably occurs more often, and has been better studied than have been the cases of female "eunuchs." The latter are women born with atresia of the ovaries (Wilkins and Fleischmann—250); their physical and emotional make-up seems to be different from that of girls who had to be castrated early. Omitting the effects of hypogonadism on the metabolism and on the body build, our concern is only with its effects upon the emotional household.

Whether the lack of gonadal stimulation shows its psycho-

logical effect in early childhood, or whether this is the result
of metabolic changes caused by the missing endocrine link,
one recognizes hypogonadism early in the little boy's personality. It is probably the persistence of a neutral, asexual form,
rather than "femininity," which gives the striking impression
of a deviation from normal boyishness. Boys with definite
gonadal deficiency do not show the characteristics of "emotional bisexuality." They are, rather, asexual. In little girls
born without ovaries, the asexuality is not as conspicuous.
Probably our expectations decide our judgment, which recognizes the passivity of the little boy as pathological, while it accepts the passive little girl's "sweetness" as normal. Probably
in girls the normal identification with the mother accounts
for a behavior which is adequately girlish. The intellectual
endowment and developmental capacity of the total personality determines the adjustment which such a child—either boy
or girl—may achieve during the prepubertal age. It seems that
this period evolves "normally"—i.e., in a way in which the
particular child would develop under the influence of his
specific environment. Puberty is the time when the hypogonadism becomes painfully obvious to the individual and
sets him apart from his group. The adaptive task of the girl
appears easier than that of male eunuchoids. This is probably
because the girl's undeveloped body and increasing shyness
do not stamp her as conspicuously unfeminine. While her
emotional life becomes deeply inhibited (constricted, in a
sense), she may go along with her companions, almost unno-
ticed. She does not become the center of hostile attention as
does the male eunuchoid. Thus the male eunuchoid's personality development after puberty is dependent upon his
capacity to adjust to his own inadequacy. This is a formidable
task, which is often made even more difficult by the unsympa-
thetic attitude of the environment, even of the boy's own family. For the family cannot react to this condition with the same
sympathy with which they would meet another inborn condi-

tion. The sense of shame which accompanies sexual failure modifies the reaction to the eunuchoid in such a way as to render his adjustment unbearably difficult. There are only a few detailed studies on the personality development and characteristics of the eunuchoids in our society. The more recent interest in their response to endocrine therapy centers mostly in the physical changes in their sex characteristics and sexual function. Carmichael (45) published a case of a eunuchoid whom he analyzed. The psychoanalysis of this man began after the testosterone propionate had produced the bodily sex characteristics which occur normally at puberty. The endocrine treatment was continued during the psychoanalysis. This patient had all the characteristic ego defenses of a severely inhibited, compulsive-neurotic personality. While his early development accounted for a severe superego, his symptoms developed mainly after the usual age of puberty, when his deficiency activated his resentment because of his "castration" as well as shame on account of his inadequacy. However, his emotions were easily hidden in the correctly regulated life of a bank clerk. His emotions were "cold" and not too disturbing, until the endocrine therapy actually stirred him up. Then he needed psychoanalytic therapy to resolve the conflicts which interfered with his adjustment to sexuality.

Daniels and Tauber (233) studied the emotional adjustment to replacement therapy after surgical castration. Their observations revealed another aspect of the psychic influences upon hormonal action. The castration, and the loss of sexual potency, represent a trauma which brought to the fore the regressive trends of those individuals; the regression in turn interfered with the willingness to continue with the therapy. Psychological factors, such as the patient's ability and willingness to experience sexual stimulation, to "put up a fight" for potency, etc., decide the effectiveness of the replacement therapy.

The influence of hypogonadism upon the integration of

sexual drive and its manifestations in sexual aspirations is well established. It remains to ask whether severe psychic traumata in early childhood could interfere with normal integration of the endocrine functions to a degree sufficient to cause hypogonadism.

Dr. Helen McLean analyzed a patient whose case is revealing.[1]

A 22-year-old woman suffered from definite hypogonadism. As a child, she had thought that she was short in comparison with other children; she began to grow when she was thirteen years old and grew even more rapidly after a visit to her home when she was sixteen. Her father and mother were of normal stature; her mother had had eight children. There are no known endocrinopathies in her family. The patient was 70 inches tall when she entered psychoanalytic therapy. She had received endocrine therapy for more than a year; however, the epiphyses of the long bones were not yet closed, and she grew another three-quarters of an inch during the first year of analysis. She was an intelligent, sensitive, and self-sacrificing girl. She suffered because she "felt" like a girl, but physically was not a girl; she had no breasts, she had never menstruated; the vaginal smears did not show ovarian activity. Her personality was markedly that of a striving, independent person, with the ambitions and givingness of a "good provider" (whether this means to be the father or the mother). She had a traumatic childhood. Her father and her older brother died when she was a baby, during the influenza epidemic in 1918. She lived with her grandmother until she was five years old; then her mother remarried and the patient lived with her mother and stepfather. The mother had six children at yearly intervals. Always pregnant and tired, she demanded of the patient that she act as a nurse for her and the babies. The patient was willing to serve, but when this involved staying away from school, she decided at ten years of age to leave home. She worked as a nursemaid for neighbors and continued her schooling. Still she felt responsible for helping the mother and went home after she finished grade school. This was about the time she first noticed her unusual growth. Later, she left her family because it was not "a good home for her" and

[1] Unpublished. I am grateful to Dr. McLean for her permission to publish this case material.

then returned again when she was sixteen and her mother had her last child. This was the last time she attempted to live there. Since then she has not lived at home, but she feels responsible for her siblings and helps them in every way. Her anger for her deprivations appears to be completely repressed. During her psychoanalytic treatment, she enjoyed the attention of a sympathetic woman doctor, an indulgence which she had never had before; she relaxed some of her burdens; she stopped growing and developed slight, irregular "spotting." This might perhaps have happened as a result of the endocrine therapy, but probably the psychoanalysis permitted her to become "more womanly."

Retrospective analysis can hardly make certain of the factors which arrested this patient's endocrine development. We should consider her strong ego-tendency to repress passive-receptive tendencies. Did this occur as a result of identification with her father and brother who died when she was one year old? Or was this the reaction to the separation from the mother, which she might have experienced as a rejection? No doubt she tried to be the helper and protector of the mother, as if she would act in her father's place. Many factors in her later childhood might have reinforced her "masculine" identification; probably the "oedipal tendencies" toward her stepfather required a concentrated effort of repression, and the need for identification with her mother was certainly discouraged by the behavior of the mother, who appeared weakened by many pregnancies, ineffectual, and demanding. Overwork and undernourishment were significant, but the emotional struggle against femininity deserves consideration also in the arresting of pituitary function.

The author analyzed an unmarried woman in her late thirties whose clinical diagnosis, for many years, had been Cushing's syndrome. She was sensitive, intuitive, and highly endowed intellectually. During analysis, she remembered a trauma with tremendously intense emotional discharge which occured when she was two years old. The exactness of the recovered memory could be verified by family photographs and by other data. The patient, without interpretation from the analyst, found that this trauma, which occurred immediately after the birth of her brother and made her ashamed, guilty, and, at the same time, boundlessly angry and helpless toward her father, caused her lasting fear of sexuality and avoidance of men.[1] Science can be satisfied only if such unusual psychoanalytic reconstructions can be validated by direct observations on the development of traumatized children.

The interaction between the organic (i.e., gonadal) factors and the psychosexual economy represents a labile equilibrium. Since the psychological side of this equilibrium is the result of sexual maturation, the reciprocal interaction between gonadal functions and emotions can be studied *longitudinally*—i.e., in the developmental history of the individual and of his symptoms. Since the equilibrium fluctuates under internal and external influences, it can also be studied in its *transverse sections*—i.e., in any selected situation.

The psychosomatic approach to the problems of sexual dysfunctions permits the construction of a series at one end of which we may place the primarily organic dysfunctions and at the other, the primarily psychologically determined conditions. Since each condition is determined by the interaction of the organic and psychic factors, neither aspect can be considered to the exclusion of the other; for they represent mutually dependent variables which sustain the sexual attitudes and functions through the range from normal to abnormal behavior.

[1] The patient died of Cushing's disease about ten months after the interruption of the analysis, which had given her much relief.

Chapter XVI

Therapy

THIS BOOK deals with the fundamental principles of the psychosomatic approach in research, diagnosis, and therapy, and no attempt is made to describe all specific therapeutic measures required in the different conditions dealt with. Only the principles of the psychosomatic approach in therapy will be discussed in this chapter and illustrated by examples.

The psychosomatic approach is more than what has been called bedside manner or medical art, more than the magnetic influence of the physician's personality on the patient, imbuing him with trust and confidence. It is based on specific knowledge of the emotional factors operating in every case and of those physiological mechanisms by which emotional factors influence the disease process. Only with this knowledge can the psychotherapy be intelligently co-ordinated with somatic measures. A general knowledge of pathology—both psychological and somatic—is the first basic requirement.

One of the most persistent errors in this field is the belief that if emotional etiology in a case has been established, somatic medical management becomes unnecessary and the patient can be turned over to a psychiatrist. This error is the reverse of the earlier misconception—namely, that if a patient has somatic symptoms, his case belongs exclusively to the domain of the physician or specialist outside of psychiatry. Progress in modern medicine consists specifically in the co-operation of the psychiatric and non-psychiatric specialists both in diagnosis and in treatment. No matter whether its etiology is of emotional nature, once there is an active ulcer in the duodenum, therapy must attempt to remedy this local lesion. Such a patient requires general medical care, dietary management, and pharmacological treatment, or even surgery (for example, sedation or specific drugs like atropin, or surgery like vagotomy, by which the connection between the central nervous system and the afflicted organs can be blocked or severed). Psychotherapy aimed at the specific emotional factors of etiological significance is a long-range project and must be coordinated with the rest of the medical management. Above all, it must be correctly timed.

The first step is to arrive at a psychosomatic diagnosis. Essentially this is a medical diagnosis which includes the complete psychiatric evaluation of the personality factors. In the light of these, the physician is able to view the medical history in the framework of the patient's life history. These psychiatric interviews are in themselves not different from the preliminary interviews which are taken at the beginning of a psychoanalytic treatment. Their technique has been developed mainly by psychoanalysts and described by Felix Deutsch; Dunbar; Fenichel, and others (61, 75, 83). Special attention is paid to the chronological sequence of the development of the symptoms on the one hand and the patient's external life situation and emotional condition on the other. Experience shows that organic symptoms in which emotional factors are of importance have a history similar to that of any psychoneurotic symptom. Emotional conflicts which the patient cannot resolve often have a disturbing influence upon vegetative functions. This is usually how the somatic symptoms make their first appearance. These first symptoms may appear in infancy, in the latency period, or during adolescence. They seldom manifest themselves for the first time in adulthood. Careful anamnestic study of these precursory, often transitory, symptoms in earlier age periods shows that they develop during times of emotional stress and disappear with the relief of the emotional tension, only to recur whenever new conflict situations arise under the vicissitudes of life. A comparison of the emotional constellation during these different flare-ups helps to establish the patient's typical pattern. For example, in the history of peptic-ulcer patients it is not unusual to find that the first upper gastrointestinal symptoms appeared in childhood, when the patient was for the first time forced to combat his dependent desires. Eating difficulty during weaning may be the very first precursory symptom; nervous vomiting in the first school days or when a teacher whom the child (after a period of initial difficulties) has finally accepted is replaced by a less sympathetic teacher. Strenuous preparation for examinations during adolescence may be the next occasion for nervous stomach symptoms, and in adult life promotion to the first responsible job. Continued exposure to dangerous and strenuous situations during the war was one of the most common precipitating factors of such symptoms. It is only very seldom that a careful anamnestic study cannot establish such precursors, not necessarily of the ulcer symptoms, but of some other manifestations in the functions of the upper gastrointestinal tract.

In certain organic symptoms, however, it is more difficult to find such physiological antecedents. Essential hypertension is usually discovered in adulthood. On the basis of psychosomatic studies one can assume, however, that a sensitivity of the vascular system to emotional stimuli might have been present long before the actual illness developed. A long period of fluctuating blood pressure in which the systolic blood pressure is from time to time elevated has been repeatedly observed in young patients under psychoanalytic care. Hypertensive patients often report a change in their behavior, a change from frequent temper tantrums to a propensity to exert more than normal control over aggressive impulses. It is quite probable that the preliminary period of fluctuating blood pressure begins sooner or later after this change in personality has taken place. Under the chronic influence of this constant emotional stimulation of the vascular system, the regulatory mechanisms gradually lose their flexibility and the blood pressure begins to remain on a higher level. Final stabilization at a high level may occur only after definite organic changes have taken place.

It is important that the physician should be familiar with all these facts in order to obtain a reliable history. Owing to the nature of anamnestic studies, the exact data of the past can seldom be obtained with full precision and reliability. The physician has to interpret the patient's recollections in the framework of his emotional development, which can usually be reconstructed with a much greater accuracy than the history of isolated symptoms and complaints. This reconstruction requires, however, a thorough knowledge of psychodynamics, just as a physical diagnosis requires an exact knowledge of anatomy, physiology, and pathology.

After a somatic and a personality diagnosis have been made in close correlation with each other, a treatment plan can be formulated. It is self-evident that in all cases in which the local symptoms require immediate care, such as a dangerously high blood pressure, bleeding ulcers, toxic symptoms in thyroid cases, or an uncontrolled hyperglycemia in the case of diabetes, the first requirement is the relief of these presenting symptoms. These acute measures have preference over the long-range psychotherapeutic measures aimed at the basic etiological factors.

It is impossible to make rigid rules as to when psychotherapy should be initiated. In a great number of cases the medical management of local symptoms and psychotherapy can be carried out simultaneously. In other cases, psychotherapy must be postponed until the patient's physiological disturbances are improved with the help of medical management. It is important to realize that penetrating psychotherapeutic measures which attack the fundamental emotional factors are apt to lead to transient increases of emotional tensions and may thus precipitate exacerbations of somatic symptoms. In all forms of the uncovering type of psychotherapy, the physician tries to re-expose the patient's ego to the original conflict situation. The experienced psychotherapist will do this only gradually, constantly gauging the ego's capacity to deal with the conflict; yet even in a well-managed psychotherapy it is unavoidable that transitory emotional conflicts arise which may aggravate somatic symptoms. Close cooperation between the psychotherapist and the medical specialist is therefore imperative. Psychotherapy conducted in such cases without the co-operation of the medical specialist must be considered as wild therapy.[1] On the other hand, the organic member of the team must constantly bear in mind that, in all cases in which the emotional factors are of causative influence, measures aimed at the local manifestations of the disease cannot achieve more than symptomatic relief. He should, therefore, fully co-operate with the psychiatrist in establishing somatic conditions under which psychotherapy can be safely conducted. A case of ulcerative colitis which I treated required co-operation in constant adjustment of medication according to the patient's emotional ups and downs during psychotherapy. Instead of interrupting psychotherapy when warning signals such as increased frequency of stools arose, sedation and an increased dosage of atropin protected the patient from the ill effects of the increased emotional tensions which occur inevitably during analysis.

In cases of ulcerative colitis the weakness of the ego has

[1] The practice of psychotherapy by laymen consequently has serious limitations, and the lay psychotherapist as an independent practitioner will, in this era of psychosomatic medicine, soon belong to the past.

been stressed by several authors (Lindemann; Daniels—141, 56, 57, 58). In our series of cases in the Chicago Institute for Psychoanalysis, this observation has been corroborated. Many of these patients have a tendency for paranoid projection; some of them belong to the group of borderline psychoses. It is therefore of primary importance that the psychotherapist gauge how far he can go in burdening the ego with uncovering repressed impulses. In many cases, superficial supportive therapy is successful in relieving symptoms, whereas deep, penetrating therapy may lead to an aggravation of the illness or may precipitate a psychotic episode. In giving supportive therapy, the physician must be aware of the fundamental conflict situation in order to assume the right approach. In many cases, helping the patient lessen his conflict over his regressive tendencies and allowing him to repudiate responsibilities without guilt feelings may stabilize the intestinal tract. This does not mean, of course, that the personality problem has been resolved. The organic disease, however, may be controlled by these relatively simple psychotherapeutic measures.

At present we know the psychodynamic background of only a few vegetative disturbances. On the map of etiological knowledge, the uncharted areas are considerably larger than the explored ones, and further psychosomatic studies are needed to fill these gaps.

It has been emphasized that in serious organic conditions it is often necessary to concentrate at first on the presenting symptoms and restrict psychotherapy to a supportive approach. No matter how important from the practical point of view such therapeutic measures may be, it must be borne in mind that the fundamental personality problems can be resolved only by consistent psychoanalytic therapy aimed at the resolution of the basic conflicts. The physician should be cognizant of the fact that this aim cannot always be realized. Organic symptoms, no matter what their origin may be, often drain ego-alien unconsicous tendencies; they are used secondarily for expression of these tendencies.[1] The organic symptoms may save the patient from developing more severe symptoms on the psychological level. Improvement of the organic symptoms, therefore, often presents a new problem for the ego: to find a new outlet for the tendencies heretofore relieved by the organic symptoms. It is not uncommon to see in ulcerative colitis cases, less frequently in peptic-ulcer patients, that improvement in the organic condition is followed by a severe exacerbation of psychological symptoms. The patient who gives expression to his urge for restitution or for hostile destructive tendencies by diarrhea is deprived of this outlet when his symptoms subside. His ego, if still unable to handle these tendencies, takes recourse to projection in the form of paranoid delusions. Similarly, when the stomach symptoms of peptic-ulcer patients improve, these patients may have to face their dependent tendencies in their original form, as the longing to receive help and love from persons on whom they are dependent. Sometimes the ego is not capable of accepting these dependent wishes and defends itself from them by projection, according to the Freudian formula, "I do not love him, I hate him—he hates me." Thus the embarrassing situation arises that the patient, relieved of his stomach symptoms, begins to show a paranoid trend which interferes with his personal relationships.

One must bear in mind that every organic symptom has an emotional significance for the patient of which his ego takes advantage for the relief of emotional conflicts. Often the mere fact of being organically ill is an important item in the emotional household of a neurotic patient. It allows regression to a more infantile dependent attitude. Curing him of his ailment creates a new problem. It increases his responsibilities, deprives him of an excuse for regression. He must then find some substitute for the emotional gap which the disappear-

---

[1] This point has been stressed by K. Menninger ("The Choice of the Lesser Evil," in *Man Against Himself*. New York, Harcourt, Brace and Company, 1938).

ance of the organic symptom has left. The patient's conscious desire to be relieved of organic symptoms cannot be taken entirely at its face value. Consciously he wants to be cured, but his neurotic needs are often better served by illness. The experienced psychotherapist, therefore, is aware of the emotional problems created by the disappearance of organic symptoms.

This double aspect of sickness—suffering and gratification of dependence—is of particular significance in our era of departmentalization of medical practice. The same patient may become cured from the point of view of the physician and remain sick from the point of view of the psychiatrist. The physician who took care of the organic side of the problem feels justified in dismissing the patient as cured, and considers the newly arisen neurotic symptoms as a distinct and independent disease, which does not come within his realm of responsibility. The psychosomatic approach calls attention to the fact that the patient's problems cannot be divided into physical and mental; they must be treated in their totality. And yet both the somatic and the psychotherapeutic approach require highly trained specialists who cannot master both techniques equally well. The only solution for this dilemma is teamwork in therapy, a close co-operation between psychiatrists and medical specialists.

It is impossible to make generalizations concerning details of the psychotherapeutic procedure. The knowledge of the central emotional conflict situations which are more or less specific in the different forms of the vegetative disturbances makes it possible for the therapist to make faster progress in the treatment.

It is often possible, for example, to relieve a patient from his asthma attacks by giving him opportunity to "confess" his repressed ego-alien tendencies in a few psychotherapeutic interviews.

The peptic-ulcer patient can sometimes be relieved from

acute symptoms within a few interviews if he is given legitimate outlets for passive dependent desires. The physician may order the patient in an authoritative manner to go on a vacation, thus giving him an acceptable excuse for relaxing. A more subtle approach is to give outlet for the patient's dependent needs in the transference situation. This can be achieved by analyzing the guilt and pride which are the emotional factors responsible for the repression of passive dependent longings, or aggressive demanding attitudes.

The hypertensive patient often improves when he feels permitted to express his pent-up, hostile impulses during the interviews or encouraged to a greater amount of self-assertion in occupational situations or in relation to his family. The analysis of guilt feelings and dependent needs in these cases contributes greatly to the patient's ability to express his self-assertive tendencies with greater freedom and to find suitable outlets for his tensions.

In the treatment of arthritis, the physician's knowledge of the specific emotional constellations may be helpful in hastening remissions. He knows that if the patient can express his resentment in conjunction with useful service to others, his symptoms often subside. The environmental conditions can often be manipulated and rendered suitable for draining hostile impulses through acceptable channels. The resulting relaxation of muscle tension may then beneficially influence the symptoms.

A more efficient co-ordination of somatic and psychotherapeutic measures is one of the great challenges confronting present-day medical science. To meet this challenge will require a more precise knowledge of the relationship of constitutional, emotional, and physiological factors in the causation of disease.

Bibliography

1. ABRAHAM, K.: "Ejaculatio Praecox," Chapter 13 in *Selected Papers*. London, Hogarth Press and Institute of Psycho-Analysis, 1927.
2. ———: "Hysterical Dream States," Chapter 4 in *Selected Papers*. London, Hogarth Press and Institute of Psycho-Analysis, 1927.
3. ———: "Manic-depressive States and the Pregenital Levels of the Libido," Chapter 26 in *Selected Papers*. London, Hogarth Press and Institute of Psycho-Analysis, 1927.
4. ———: "The Spending of Money in Anxiety States," Chapter 14, in *Selected Papers*. London, Hogarth Press and Institute of Psycho-Analysis, 1927.
5. ABRAMSON, D. I.: *Vascular Responses in the Extremities of Man in Health and Disease*. Chicago, University of Chicago Press, 1944.
6. ACKERMAN, N. W., and CHIDESTER, L.: " 'Accidental' Self-Injury in Children," *Arch. Pediat.* 53:711, 1936.
7. ALEXANDER, F.: "Emotional Factors in Essential Hypertension," *Psychosom. Med.* 1:173, 1939.
8. ———: *Fundamentals of Psychoanalysis*. New York, W. W. Norton & Company, Inc., 1948.
9. ———: "The Influence of Psychologic Factors upon Gastro-intestinal Disturbances: A Symposium. I. General Principles, Objectives and Preliminary Results," *Psychoanalyt. Quart.* 3:501, 1934.
10. ———: *The Medical Value of Psychoanalysis*. New York, W. W. Norton & Company, Inc., 1936.

11. ———: "Psychoanalytic Study of a Case of Essential Hypertension," *Psychosom. Med.* 1:139, 1939.

12. ———: "Training Principles in Psychosomatic Medicine," *Am. J. Orthopsychiat.* 16:410, 1946.

13. ———: "Treatment of a Case of Peptic Ulcer and Personality Disorder," *Psychosom. Med.* 9:320, 1947.

14. ALEXANDER, F., *et al.*: "The Influence of Psychologic Factors Upon Gastro-intestinal Disturbances: A Symposium. *Psychoanalyt. Quart.* 3:501, 1934.

15. ALEXANDER, F., and MENNINGER, W. C.: Relation of Persecutory Delusions to the Functioning of the Gastro-intestinal Tract," *J. Nerv. & Ment. Dis.* 84:541, 1936.

16. ALEXANDER, F., and PORTIS, S. A.: "A Psychosomatic Study of Hypoglycaemic Fatigue," *Psychosom. Med.* 6:191, 1944.

17. ALKAN, L.: *Anatomische Organkrankheiten aus seelischer Ursache.* Stuttgart und Leipzig, Hippokrates-Verlag, 1930.

18. ALVAREZ, W. C.: *Nervous Indigestion.* New York, P. B. Hoeber, Inc., 1930.

19. ———: "Ways in Which Emotion Can Affect the Digestive Tract," *J.A.M.A.*, 92:1231, 1929.

20. BACON, C.: "The Influence of Psychologic Factors upon Gastro-Intestinal Disturbances: A Symposium. II. Typical Personality Trends and Conflicts in Cases of Gastric Disturbance," *Psychoanalyt. Quart.* 3:540, 1934.

21. BALZAC, H. de: *Cousin Pons.* New York, The Century Co. 1906.

22. BARATH, E.: "Arterial Hypertension and Physical Work," *Arch. Int. Med.* 42:297, 1928.

23. BARTEMEIER, L. H.: "A Psychoanalytic Study of a Case of Chronic Exudative Dermatitis," *Psychoanalyt. Quart.* 7:216, 1938.

24. BEACH, F. A.: *Hormones and Behavior.* New York and London, Paul B. Hoeber, Inc., 1948.

25. BENEDEK, T.: "Climacterium: a Developmental Phase." (To be published in the *Psychoanalytic Quarterly.*)

26. ———: "The Psychosomatic Implications of the Primary Unit: Mother-Child," *Am. J. Orthopsychiat.* 19:642, 1949.

27. ———: "Die ueberwertige Idee und ihre Beziehung zur Suchtkrankheit," *Internat. Ztschr. f. Psychoanal.* 22:59, 1936.

28. BENEDEK, T., and RUBENSTEIN, B. B.: *The Sexual Cycle in Women.* Psychosom. Med. Monographs, Volume III, Nos. I and II. Washington, D.C., National Research Council, 1942.

29. BENJAMIN, J. D., COLEMAN, J. V., and HORNBEIN, R.: "A Study of Personality in Pulmonary Tuberculosis," *Am. J. Orthopsychiat.* 18:704, 1948.

30. BERGMANN, G. VON: "Ulcus duodeni und vegetatives Nervensystem," *Berliner Klinische Wchnschr.* 50:2374, 1913.

31. ——: "Zum Abbau der 'Organneurosen' als Folge Interner Diagnostik," *Deutsche Med. Wchnschr.*, Leipzig, Vol. 53, No. 49, p. 2057, 1927.

32. BINGER, C. A. L., ACKERMAN, N. W., COHN, A. E., SCHROEDER, H. A., and STEELE, J. H.: *Personality in Arterial Hypertension.* New York, American Society for Research in Psychosomatic Problems, 1945.

33. BOND, E.: "Psychiatric Contributions to the Study of the Gastrointestinal System," *Am. J. Digest. Dis.* 5:482, 1938.

34. BOOTH, G. C.: "The Psychological Approach in Therapy of Chronic Arthritis," *Rheumatism* Vol. 1, No. 3, p. 48, 1939.

35. BRADLEY, S. E.: "Physiology of Essential Hypertension," *Am. J. Med.* 4:398, 1948.

36. BRENNER, C., FRIEDMAN, A. P., and CARTER, S.: "Psychologic Factors in the Etiology and Treatment of Chronic Headache," *Psychosom. Med.* 11:53, 1949.

37. BROH-KAHN, R. H., PODORE, C. J., and MIRSKY, I. A.: "Uropepsin Excretion by Man. II. Uropepsin Excretion by Healthy Men," *J. Clin. Investigation* 27:825, 1948.

38. BRAM, I.: "Psychic Trauma in Pathogenesis of Exophthalmic Goiter," *Endocrinology* 11:106, 1927.

39. BROWN, W. L.: "Biology of the Endocrine System," *New York Med. J.* 115:373, 1922.

40. BROWN, W. T., and GILDEA, E. A.: "Hyperthyroidism and Personality," *Am. J. Psychiat.* 94:59, 1937.

41. BROWN, W. T., PREU, P. W., and SULLIVAN, A. J.: "Ulcerative Colitis and the Personality," *Am. J. Psychiat.* 95:407, 1938.

42. BRUCH, H., and HEWELETT, E.: "Psychologic Aspects of the Medical Management of Diabetes in Children," *Psychosom. Med.* 9:205, 1947.

43. CANNON, W. B.: *Bodily Changes in Pain, Hunger, Fear and Rage.* Second Edition. New York, D. Appleton & Co., 1920.

44. CARLSON, H. B., McCULLOCH, W., and ALEXANDER, F.: "Effects of Zest on Blood Sugar Regulation." Read by title at the A. Research Nerv. & Ment. Dis., New York, December 9, 1949.

45. CARMICHAEL, H. T.: "A Psychoanalytic Study of a Case of Eunuchoidism," *Psychoanalyt. Quart.* 10:243, 1941.

46. CHADWICK, M.: *The Psychological Effects of Menstruation.* Nerv. & Ment. Dis. Monograph Series No. 56. New York and Washington, Nerv. & Ment. Dis. Publ. Co., 1932.

47. CLARK, D., HOUGH, H., and WOLFF, H. G.: "Experimental Studies on Headache. Observations on Histamine Headache," *A. Research Nerv. & Ment. Dis. Proc.* 15:417, 1935.

48. COLWELL, A. R.: "Observed Course of Diabetes Mellitus and Inferences Concerning its Origin and Progress," *Arch. Int. Med.* 70:523, 1942.

49. CONRAD, A.: "The Psychiatric Study of Hyperthyroid Patients," *J. Nerv. & Ment. Dis.* 79:505, 1934.

50. CORIAT, I.: "Sex and Hunger," *Psychoanalyt. Rev.* 8:375, 1921.

51. CORMIA, F., and SLIGHT, D.: "Psychogenic Factors in Dermatoses," *Canad. M. A. J.* 33:527, 1935.

52. CRILE, G.: "The Mechanism of Exophthalmic Goitre," Third Int. Goitre Conf. and Am. A. for the Study of Goitre. Proc. 1938, p. 1.

53. CSERNA, I.: "Adatok az Icterus Neonatorum Tanahoz," *Orvosi hetil,* 67:42.

54. DALE, H. H., and FELDBERG, W.: "Chemical Transmitter of Vagus Effects to Stomach," *J. Physiol.* 81:320, 1934.

55. DANIELS, G. E.: "Analysis of a Case of Neurosis with Diabetes Mellitus," *Psychoanalyt. Quart.* 5:513, 1936.

56. ———: "Psychiatric Aspects of Ulcerative Colitis," *New England J. Med.* 226:178, 1942.

57. ———: "Psychiatric Factors in Ulcerative Colitis," *Gastroenterology* 10:59, 1948.

58. ———: "Treatment of a Case of Ulcerative Colitis Associated with Hysterical Depression," *Psychosom. Med.* 2:276, 1940.

59. DARWIN, C. R.: *The Expression of the Emotions in Man and Animals.* London, J. Murray, 1872.

60. DE ROBERTIS, E.: "Assay of Thyrotropic Hormone in Human Blood," *J. Clin. Endocrinol.* 8:956, 1948.

61. DEUTSCH, F.: "Associative Anamnesis," *Psychoanalyt. Quart.* 8:354, 1939.

62. DEUTSCH, F., and NADELL, R.: "Psychosomatic Aspects of Dermatology with Special Consideration of Allergic Phenomena," *Nerv. Child* 5:339, 1946.

63. DEUTSCH, H.: *The Psychology of Women,* Vols. I and II. New York, Grune & Stratton, 1944, 1945.

64. DRAGSTEDT, L. R.: "Section of the Vagus Nerves to the Stomach in the Treatment of Peptic Ulcer," *Surg., Gynec. & Obst.* 83:547, 1946.

65. ———: "Some Physiological Principles in Surgery of the Stomach," *Canad. M. A. J.* 56:133, 1947.

66. DRAGSTEDT, L. R., and OWENS, F. M., Jr.: "Supradiaphragmatic Section of Vagus Nerves in Treatment of Duodenal Ulcer," *Proc. Soc. Exper. Biol. & Med.* 53:152, 1943.

67. DRAPER, G.: "The Common Denominator of Disease," *Am. J. M. Sc.* 190:545, 1935.

68. ———: "The Emotional Component of the Ulcer Susceptible Constitution," *Ann. Int. Med.* 16:633, 1942.

69. ———: *Human Constitution; a Consideration of its Relationship to Disease.* Philadelphia & London, W. B. Saunders Company, 1924.

70. DRAPER, G., and TOURAINE, G. A.: "The Man-Environment Unit and Peptic Ulcer," *Arch. Int. Med.* 49:616, 1932.

71. DUNBAR, F.: *Emotions and Bodily Changes.* Third Edition. New York, Columbia University Press, 1947.

72. ———: *Mind and Body: Psychosomatic Medicine.* New York, Random House, 1947.

73. ———: "Physical Mental Relationships in Illness; Trends in Modern Medicine and Research as Related to Psychiatry," *Am. J. Psychiat.* 91:541, 1934.

74. ———: "Psychoanalytic Notes Relating to Syndromes of Asthma and Hay Fever," *Psychoanalyt. Quart.* 7:25, 1938.

75. ———: *Psychosomatic Diagnosis.* New York, London, Paul B. Hoeber, Inc., 1943.

76. EINSTEIN, A., and INFELD, L.: *The Evolution of Physics.* New York, Simon & Schuster, 1938.

77. EISENBUD, J.: "The Psychology of Headache," *Psychiat. Quart.* 11:592, 1937.

78. ENGEL, G. L., FERRIS, E. B., and ROMANO, J.: "Studies of Syncope," *Cincinnati J. Med.* 26:93, 1945.

79. ENGEL, G. L., and ROMANO, J.: "Studies of Syncope: IV. Biologic Interpretation of Vasodepressor Syncope," *Psychosom. Med.* 9:288, 1947.

80. ENGEL, G. L., ROMANO, J., and McLIN, T. R.: "Vasodepressor and Carotid Sinus Syncope. Clinical, Electroencephalographic

and Electrocardiographic Observations," *Arch. Int. Med.* 74:100, 1944.

81. FAHRENKAMP, K.: *Die psychophysischen Wechselwirkungen bei den Hypertonie-erkrankungen.* Stuttgart, Hippokrates-Verlag, 1926.

82. FARQUHARSON, H., and HYLAND, H. H.: "Anorexia Nervosa," *J.A.M.A.* 111:1085, 1938.

83. FENICHEL, O.: *The Psychoanalytic Theory of Neurosis.* New York, W. W. Norton & Company, Inc., 1945.

84. FERENCZI, S.: "Disease- or Patho-Neuroses," Chapter 5 in *Further Contributions to the Theory and Technique of Psychoanalysis.* London, Hogarth Press and the Institute of Psycho-Analysis, 1926.

85. FERRIS, E. B., REISER, M. F., STEAD, W. W., and BRUST, A. A., JR.: "Clinical and Physiological Observations of Interrelated Mechanisms in Arterial Hypertension," *Trans. A. Am. Physicians* 61:97, 1948.

86. FICARRA, B. J., and NELSON, R. A.: "Phobia as a Symptom in Hyperthyroidism," *Am. J. Psychiat.* 103:831, 1947.

87. FISHBERG, A. M.: *Hypertension and Nephritis.* Third edition. Philadelphia, Lea and Febiger, 1934.

88. FRENCH, T. M.: "Physiology of Behavior and Choice of Neurosis," *Psychoanalyt. Quart.* 10:561, 1941.

89. FRENCH, T. M., ALEXANDER, F., et al.: *Psychogenic Factors in Bronchial Asthma,* Parts I and II. Psychosom. Med. Monographs IV, and II, Nos. I and II. Washington, National Research Council, 1941.

90. FRENCH, T. M., in collaboration with JOHNSON, A. M.: "Brief Psychotherapy in Bronchial Asthma," in *Proceedings of the Second Brief Psychotherapy Council.* Chicago, Institute for Psychoanalysis, 1944.

91. FRENCH, T. M., and SHAPIRO, L. B.: "The Use of Dream Analysis in Psychosomatic Research." *Psychosom. Med.* 11:110, 1949.

92. FREUD, S.: "The Justification for Detaching from Neurasthenia a Particular Syndrome: the Anxiety-Neurosis," Chapter 5 in *Collected Papers,* Vol. I. Second Edition. London, Hogarth Press and the Institute of Psycho-Analysis, 1940.

93. ———: "Mourning and Melancholia," Chapter 8 in *Collected Papers,* Vol. IV. Third Edition. London, Hogarth Press and the Institute of Psycho-Analysis, 1946.

94. ———: *Three Contributions to the Theory of Sex*. Nerv. & Ment. Dis. Monograph Series No. 7. New York and Washington, Nerv. & Ment. Dis. Publ. Co., 1930.

95. ———: *Wit and Its Relation to the Unconscious*. New York, Moffat, Yard, 1916.

96. FROMM-REICHMANN, F.: "Contribution to the Psychogenesis of Migraine," *Psychoanalyt. Rev.* 24:26, 1937.

97. GASKELL, W. H.: *Origin of Vertebrates*. New York, Longmans, Green & Co., 1908.

98. ———: "Phylogenetic considerations," *Brit. M.J.* 1:720, 1886.

99. GERARD, M. W.: "Enuresis. A Study in Etiology," *Am. J. Orthopsychiat.* 9:48, 1939.

100. GILLESPIE, R. D.: "Psychological Aspects of Skin Diseases," *Brit. J. Dermat.* 50:1, 1938.

101. GOLDBLATT, H.: "Studies on Experimental Hypertension. V. The Pathogenesis of Experimental Hypertension Due to Renal Ischemia," *Ann. Int. Med.* 11:69, 1937.

102. GOLDSCHEIDER, K.: *Ztschr. f. aerztl. Fortbildung*, Vol. 23, No. 1, Seite 1, 1926 (quoted from Fahrenkamp).

103. GOODALL, J. S., and ROGERS, L.: "The Effects of the Emotions in the Production of Thyrotoxicosis," *M. J. & Rec.* 138:411, 1933.

104. GRAHAM, J. R., and WOLFF, H. G.: "Mechanism of Migraine Headache and Action of Ergotamine Tartrate," *Arch. Neurol. & Psychiat.* 39:737, 1938.

105. GREGG, A.: "The Future of Medicine," *Harvard Medical Alumni Bulletin*, Cambridge. Vol. 11 (October, 1936).

106. GROEN, J.: "Psychogenesis and Psychotherapy of Ulcerative Colitis," *Psychosom. Med.* 9:151, 1947.

107. GULL, W.: "Anorexia Nervosa," *Tr. Clin. Soc.*, London, 7:22, 1874.

108. GUTHEIL, E.: "Analysis of a Case of Migraine," *Psychoanalyt. Rev.* 21:272, 1934.

109. HALLIDAY, J. L.: "Approach to Asthma," *Brit. J. M. Psychol.* 17:1, 1937.

110. ———: "Concept of a Psychosomatic Affection," *Lancet*, London, 2:692, 1943.

111. ———: "Epidemiology and the Psychosomatic Affections; a Study in Social Medicine," *Lancet*, London, 2:185, 1946.

112. ———: "The Incidence of Psychosomatic Affections in Britain," *Psychosom. Med.* 7:135, 1945.

113. ———: "Psychological Aspects of Rheumatoid Arthritis," *Proc. Roy. Soc. Med.* 35:455, 1942.

114. ———: "Psychological Factors in Rheumatism: Preliminary Study," *Brit. M. J.* 1:213, 264, 1937.

115. ———: *Psychosocial Medicine. A Study of the Sick Society.* New York, W. W. Norton & Company, Inc., 1948.

116. HAM, G. C., ALEXANDER, F., and CARMICHAEL, H. T.: "Dynamic Aspects of the Personality Features and Reactions Characteristic of Patients with Graves' Disease." Presented at the A. Research Nerv. & Ment. Dis., New York, December 9, 1949.

117. HARTMAN, H. R.: "Neurogenic Factors in Peptic Ulcer," *M. Clin. North America* 16:1357, 1933.

118. HILL, L. B.: "A Psychoanalytic Observation on Essential Hypertension," *Psychoanalyt. Rev.* 22:60, 1935.

119. HIMWICH, H. E.: "A Review of Hypoglycemia, Its Physiology and Pathology, Symptomatology and Treatment," *Am. J. Digest. Dis.* 11:1, 1944.

120. HINKLE, L. E., CONGER, G. A., and WOLF, S.: "Experimental Evidence on the Mechanism of Diabetic Ketosis," *J. Clin. Investigation* 28:788, 1949.

121. HINKLE, L. E., and WOLF, S.: "Experimental Study of Life Situations, Emotions, and the Occurrence of Acidosis in a Juvenile Diabetic," *Am. J. M. Sc.* 217:130, 1949.

122. HOSKINS, R. G.: *Endocrinology.* Revised Edition. New York, W. W. Norton & Company, Inc., 1950.

123. JACKSON, D. D.: "The Psychosomatic Factors in Ulcerative Colitis," *Psychosom. Med.* 8:278, 1946.

124. JELLIFFE, S. E., and EVANS, E.: "Psoriasis as an Hysterical Conversion Symbolization," *New York Med. J.* 104:1077, 1916.

125. JOHNSON, A. M.: "A Case of Migraine," in *Proceedings of the Third Psychotherapy Council.* Chicago, Institute for Psychoanalysis, 1946.

126. JOHNSON, A. M., SHAPIRO, L. B., and ALEXANDER, F.: "A Preliminary Report on a Psychosomatic Study of Rheumatoid Arthritis," *Psychosom. Med.* 9:295, 1947.

127. JONES, E.: "Urethralerotik und Ehrgeiz," *Internatl. Ztschr. f. Aerztl. Psychoanal.* 3:156, 1915.

128. JOSLIN, E. P., ROOT, H. F., WHITE, P., MARBLE, A., and BAILEY, C. C.: *The Treatment of Diabetes Mellitus.* Eighth Edition. Philadelphia, Lea and Febiger, 1947.

129. KAPP, F. T., ROSENBAUM, M., and ROMANO, J.: "Psychological Factors in Men with Peptic Ulcers," *Am. J. Psychiat.* 103:700, 1947.

130. KEPECS, J., ROBIN, M., and BRUNNER, M. J.: "The Relationship of Certain Emotional States and Transudation into the Skin." Presented at the Annual Meeting of the Am. Psychosom. Soc. Atlantic City, April 30, 1949.

131. KING, E. L., and HERRING, J. S.: "Hypothyroidism in the Causation of Abortion, Especially of the 'Missed' Variety," *J.A.M.A.* 113:1300, 1939.

132. KLAUDER, J. V.: "Psychogenic Aspects of Diseases of the Skin," *Arch. Neurol. & Psychiat.* 33:221, 1935.

133. KNOPF, O.: "Preliminary Report on Personality Studies in 30 Migraine Patients," *J. Nerv. & Ment. Dis.* 82:270, 400, 1935.

134. KRONFELD, A.: "Oesophagus-Neurosen," *Psychotherapeut. Praxis* 1:21, 1934.

135. LASÉGUE, C.: "On Hysterical Anorexia," *Med. Times and Gaz.* 2:265, 1873.

136. LEVEY, H. B.: "The Influence of Psychologic Factors upon Gastro-Intestinal Disturbances. A Symposium. IV. Oral Trends and Oral Conflicts in a Case of Duodenal Ulcer," *Psychoanalyt. Quart.* 3:574, 1934.

137. LEVINE, M.: "The Influence of Psychologic Factors upon Gastro-Intestinal Disturbances. A Symposium. V. Pregenital Trends in a Case of Chronic Diarrhea and Vomiting," *Psychoanalyt. Quart.* 3:583, 1934.

138. LEWIS, N. D. C.: "Psychoanalytic Study of Hyperthyroidism," *Psychoanalyt. Rev.* 10:140, 1923.

139. ———: "Psychological Factors in Hyperthyroidism," *M. J. & Rec.* 122:121, 1925.

140. LIDZ, T.: "Emotional Factors in the Etiology of Hyperthyroidism," *Psychosom. Med.* 11:2, 1949.

141. LINDEMANN, E.: "Psychiatric Problems in Conservative Treatment of Ulcerative Colitis," *Arch. Neurol. & Psychiat.* 53:322, 1945.

142. LONG, C. N. H.: "Conditions Associated with Secretion of Adrenal Cortex," *Federation Proc.* 6:461, 1947.

143. LORAND, S.: "Psychogenic Factors in a Case of Angioneurotic Edema," *J. Mt. Sinai Hosp.* 2:231, 1936.

144. MAHL, G. F.: "Effect of Chronic Fear on the Gastric Secretion of HCL in Dogs," *Psychosom. Med.* 11:30, 1949.

145. MARAÑON, G.: "Le facteur émotionnel dans la pathogénie des étâts hyperthyroïdiens," *Ann. méd.* 9:81, 1921.
146. MARBE, K.: *Praktische Psychologie der Unfaelle und Betriebsschaeden.* Muenchen-Berlin, R. Oldenbourg, 1926.
147. MARCUSSEN, R. M., and WOLFF, H. G.: "Therapy of Migraine," *J.A.M.A.* 139:198, 1949.
148. MARKEE, J. E., SAWYER, C. H., and HOLLINSHEAD, W. H.: "Andrenergic Control of the Release of Luteinizing Hormone from the Hypophysis of the Rabbit," *Recent Progr. Hormone Research* 2:117, 1948.
149. MASLOW, A.: "The Role of Dominance in the Social and Sexual Behavior of Infra-Human Primates: III. A Theory of Sexual Behavior of Infra-Human Primates," *J. Genet. Psychol.* 48:310, 1936.
150. MEYER, A., BOLLMEIER, L. N., and ALEXANDER, F.: "Correlation between Emotions and Carbohydrate Metabolism in Two Cases of Diabetes Mellitus," *Psychosom. Med.* 7:335, 1945.
151. MEAD, M.: *Male and Female.* New York, William Morrow & Company, 1949.
152. MENNINGER, K.: "Emotional Factors in Hypertension," *Bull. Menninger Clin.* 2:74, 1938.
153. ———: "Polysurgery and Polysurgical Addiction," *Psychoanalyt. Quart.* 3:173, 1934.
154. MENNINGER, K., and MENNINGER, W. C.: "Psychoanalytic Observations in Cardiac Disorders," *Am. Heart J.* 11:10, 1936.
155. MEYER, K., PRUDDEN, J. F., LEHMAN, W. L., and STEINBERG, A.: "Lysozyme Activity in Ulcerative Alimentary Disease. I. Lysozyme in Peptic Ulcer," *Am. J. Med.* 5:482, 1948.
156. MEYER, K., GELLHORN, A., PRUDDEN, J. F., LEHMAN, W. L., and STEINBERG, A.: "Lysozyme Activity in Ulcerative Alimentary Disease. II. Lysozyme Activity in Chronic Ulcerative Colitis," *Am. J. Med.* 5:496, 1948.
157. MILLER, M. L.: "Psychodynamic Mechanisms in a Case of Neurodermatitis," *Psychosom. Med.* 10:309, 1948.
158. ———: "A Psychological Study of a Case of Eczema and a Case of Neurodermatitis," *Psychosom. Med.* 4:82, 1942.
159. MIRSKY, I. A.: "Emotional Factors in the Patient with Diabetes Mellitus," *Bull. Menninger Clin.* 12:187, 1948.
160. ———: "Emotional Hyperglycemia," *Proc. Central Soc. Clin. Research* 19:74, 1946.

161. ———: "The Etiology of Diabetic Acidosis," *J.A.M.A.* 118: 690, 1942.
162. ———: "Some Considerations of the Etiology of Diabetes Mellitus in Man," *Proc. Am. Diab. A.* 5:117, 1945.
163. MIRSKY, I. A., BLOCK, S., OSHER, S., and BROH-KAHN, R. H.: "Uropepsin Excretion by Man; I. The Source, Properties and Assay of Uropepsin," *J. Clin. Investigation* 27:818, 1948.
164. MITTELMANN, B.: "Psychogenic Factors and Psychotherapy in Hyperthyreosis and Rapid Heart Imbalance," *J. Nerv. & Ment. Dis.* 77:465, 1933.
165. MITTELMANN, B., and WOLFF, H. G.: "Emotions and Gastroduodenal Function: Experimental Studies on Patients with Gastritis, Duodenitis and Peptic Ulcer," *Psychosom. Med.* 4:5, 1942.
166. MOHR, F.: *Psychophysische Behandlungsmethoden.* Leipzig, Hirzel, 1925.
167. MONTAGU, M. F. ASHLEY: *Adolescent Sterility.* Springfield, Charles C. Thomas, 1946.
168. MOSCHCOWITZ, E.: *Biology of Disease.* Mt. Sinai Hospital Monograph No. 1. New York, Grune & Stratton, 1948.
169. ———: "Hypertension: Its Significance, Relation to Arteriosclerosis and Nephritis and Etiology," *Am. J. M. Sc.* 158:668, 1919.
170. ———: "The Nature of Graves' Disease," *Arch. Int. Med.* 46:610, 1930.
171. *Motor Vehicle Traffic Conditions in the U.S.* Part 6, p. 4. 75th Congress, 3rd Session, House Document 462, Part 6, Washington, D.C., 1938.
172. MUELLER, O.: *Die Kapillaren der Menschlichen Koerperoberflaeche in Gesunden und Kranken Tagen.* Stuttgart, Ferdinand Enke, 1922.
173. MURRAY, C. D.: "A Brief Psychological Analysis of a Patient with Ulcerative Colitis," *J. Nerv. & Ment. Dis.* 72:617, 1930.
174. ———: "Psychogenic Factors in the Etiology of Ulcerative Colitis and Bloody Diarrhea," *Am. J. M. Sc.* 180:239, 1930.
175. NECHELES, H.: "A Theory on Formation of Peptic Ulcer," *Am. J. Digest. Dis. and Nutrition* 4:643, 1937.
176. ORR, D.: "Pregnancy Following the Decision to Adopt," *Psychosom. Med.* 3:441, 1941.
177. PAGE, I. H., and CORCORAN, A. C.: *Arterial Hypertension.* Chicago, The Year Book Publishers, 1945.

178. PALMER, W. L.: "Fundamental Difficulties in the Treatment of Peptic Ulcer," *J.A.M.A.* 101:1604, 1933.
179. PERLOFF, W. H.: "Role of the Hormones in Human Sexuality," *Psychosom. Med.* 11:133, 1949.
180. PODORE, C. J., BROH-KAHN, R. H., and MIRSKY, I. A.: "Uropepsin Excretion by Man. III. Uropepsin Excretion by Patients with Peptic Ulcer and Other Lesions of the Stomach," *J. Clin. Investigation* 27:834, 1948.
181. PORTIS, S. A.: "Idiopathic Ulcerative Colitis; Newer Concepts Concerning Its Cause and Management." *J.A.M.A.* 139:208, 1949.
182. PORTIS, S. A., and ZITMAN, I. H.: "A Mechanism of Fatigue in Neuro-psychiatric Patients," *J.A.M.A.* 121:569, 1943.
183. PRATT, J. P.: "Sex Functions in Man," Chapter 24 in *Sex and Internal Secretions*. Edited by E. Allen. Second Edition. Baltimore, The Williams and Wilkins Company, 1939.
184. RAHMAN, L., RICHARDSON, H. B., and RIPLEY, H. S.: "Anorexia Nervosa with Psychiatric Observations," *Psychosom. Med.* 1:335, 1939.
185. RAWSON, A. T.: "Accident Proneness," *Psychosom. Med.* 6:88, 1944.
186. RENNIE, T. A. C., and HOWARD, J. E.: "Hypoglycemia and Tension-Depression," *Psychosom. Med.* 4:273, 1942.
187. RICHARDSON, H. B.: "Simmonds' Disease and Anorexia Nervosa," *Arch. Int. Med.* 63:1, 1939.
188. RICHTER, K. M.: "Some New Observations Bearing on the Effect of Hyperthyroidism on Genital Structure and Function," *J. Morphol.* 74:375, 1944.
189. RISEMAN, J. E. F., and WEISS, S.: "Symptomatology of Arterial Hypertension," *Am. J. M. Sc.* 180:47, 1930.
190. ROMANO, J., and COON, G. P.: "Physiologic and Psychologic Studies in Spontaneous Hypoglycemia," *Psychosom. Med.* 4:283, 1942.
191. ROMANO, J., and ENGEL, G. L.: "Studies of Syncope. III. The Differentiation between Vasodepressor Syncope and Hysterical Fainting," *Psychosom. Med.* 7:3, 1945.
192. ROMANO, J., ENGEL, G. L., WEBB, J. P., FERRIS, E. B., RYDER, H. W., and BLANKENHORN, M. A.: "Syncopal Reactions during Simulated Exposure to High Altitude in Decompression Chamber," *War Med.* 4:475, 1943.
193. ROSEN, H., and LIDZ, T.: "Emotional Factors in the Precipi-

tation of Recurrent Diabetic Acidosis," *Psychosom. Med.* 11:211, 1949.

194. ROSENBAUM, M.: "Psychogenic Headache," *Cincinnati J. Med.* 28:7, 1947.

195. ROSENBAUM, M., and KAPP, F. T.: "Psychosomatic Conference of the Cincinnati General Hospital. Case No. 141, Ulcerative Colitis," *Dis. Nerv. System* 8:345, 1947.

196. ROSS, W. D.: "The Person with Ulcerative Colitis," *Canad. M.A.J.* 58:326, 1948.

197. RUBENSTEIN, B. B.: "Functional Sterility in Women," *Ohio State M.J.* 35:1066, 1939.

198. ———: "The Vaginal Smear-Basal Body Temperature Technic and Its Application to the Study of Functional Sterility in Women," *Endocrinology* 27:843, 1940.

199. RUESCH, J., CHRISTIANSEN, C., HARRIS, R. E., DEWEES, S., JACOBSON, A., and LOEB, M. B.: *Duodenal Ulcer. A Sociopsychological Study of Naval Enlisted Personnel and Civilians.* Berkeley and Los Angeles, University of California Press, 1948.

200. RUESCH, J., CHRISTIANSEN, C., PATTERSON, L. C., DEWEES, S., JACOBSON, A., in cooperation with SOLEY, M. H.: "Psychological Invalidism in Thyroidectomized Patients," *Psychosom. Med.* 9:77, 1947.

201. SADGER, J.: "Ueber sexualsymbolische Verwertung des Kopfschmerzes," *Zentralbl. f. Psychoanal.* 2:190, 1911/12.

202. SAUL, L. J.: "Hostility in Cases of Essential Hypertension," *Psychosom. Med.* 1:153, 1939.

203. SAUL, L. J., and BERNSTEIN, C.: "The Emotional Settings of Some Attacks of Urticaria," *Psychosom. Med.* 3:349, 1941.

204. SAWYER, C. H., MARKEE, J. E., and TOWNSEND, B. F.: "Cholinergic and Andrenergic Components in the Neurohumoral Control of the Release of LH in the Rabbit," *Endocrinology* 44:18, 1949.

205. SCARBOROUGH, L. F.: "Neuro-Dermatitis from a Psychosomatic Viewpoint," *Dis. Nerv. System* 9:90, 1948.

206. SCHIELE, B. C., and BROZEK, J.: " 'Experimental Neurosis' Resulting from Semistarvation in Man," *Psychosom. Med.* 10:31, 1948.

207. SCHMIED, M.: "Esstoerung und Verstimmung vor dem dritten Lebensjahr," *Ztschr. f. Psychoanal. Paed.* 10:241, 1936.

208. SCHULZE, V. E., and SCHWAB, E. H.: "Arteriolar Hypertension in the American Negro," *Am. Heart J.* 11:66, 1936.

209. SEIDENBERG, R.: "Psychosexual Headache," *Psychiat. Quart.* 21:351, 1947.
210. SELINSKY, H.: "Psychological Study of the Migrainous Syndrome," *Bull. New York Acad. Med.* 15:757, 1939.
211. SELYE, H.: "The General Adaptation Syndrome and the Diseases of Adaptation," *J. Clin. Endocrinol.* 6:117, 1946.
212. SILBERMANN, I. S.: "Experimentelle Magen-Duodenalulcuserzeugung durch Scheinfuettern nach Pavlov," *Zentralbl. f. Chir.* 54:2385, 1927.
213. SMITH, H. W.: *Lectures on the Kidney.* Lawrence, University of Kansas Press, 1943.
214. SMITH, H. W., GOLDRING, W., and CHASIS, H.: "Role of the Kidney in the Genesis of Hypertension," *Bull. New York Acad. Med.* 19:449, 1943.
215. SOFFER, L. J., VOLTERRA, M., GABRILOVE, J. L., POLLACK, A., and JACOBS, M.: "Effect of Iodine and Adrenalin on Thyrotropin in Graves' Disease and in Normal and Thyroidectomized Dogs," *Proc. Soc. Exper. Biol. & Med.* 64:446, 1947.
216. SOSKIN, S., and LEVINE, R.: *Carbohydrate Metabolism.* Chicago, University of Chicago Press, 1946.
217. SOULE, S. D.: "A Study of Thyroid Activity in Normal Pregnancy," *Am. J. Obst. & Gynec.* 23:165, 1932.
218. SPERLING, M.: "Psychoanalytic Study of Ulcerative Colitis in Children," *Psychoanalyt. Quart.* 15:302, 1946.
219. SQUIER, R., and DUNBAR, F.: "Emotional Factors in the Course of Pregnancy," *Psychosom. Med.* 7:161, 1946.
220. STOKES, J. H.: "The Nervous and Mental Component in Cutaneous Disease," *Pennsylvania M.J.* 35:229, 1932.
221. STOKES, J. H., and BEERMAN, H.: "Psychosomatic Correlations in Allergic Conditions: a Review of Problems and Literature," *Psychosom. Med.* 2:438, 1940.
222. SULLIVAN, A. J., and CHANDLER, C. A.: "Ulcerative Colitis of Psychogenic Origin," *Yale J. Biol. & Med.* 4:779, 1932.
223. SZASZ, T. S.: "Factors in the Pathogenesis of Peptic Ulcer," *Psychosom. Med.* 11:300, 1949.
224. ———: "Psychosomatic Aspects of Salivary Activity. I. Hypersalivation in Patients with Peptic Ulcer." (To be published in *Proc. of the A. for Research in Nerv. & Ment. Dis.*)
225. ———: "Psychosomatic Aspects of Salivary Activity. II. Psychoanalytic Observations Concerning Hypersalivation." (To be published.)

226. ———: "Psychiatric Aspects of Vagotomy. A Preliminary Report," *Ann. Int. Med.* 28:279, 1948.

227. ———: "Psychiatric Aspects of Vagotomy. II. A Psychiatric Study of Vagotomized Ulcer Patients with Comments on Prognosis," *Psychosom. Med.* 11:187, 1949.

228. ———: "Psychiatric Aspects of Vagotomy. III. The Problem of Diarrhea after Vagotomy." (To be published in *J. Nerv. & Ment. Dis.*)

229. ———: "Psychiatric Aspects of Vagotomy. IV. Phantom Ulcer Pain," *Arch. Neurol. & Psychiat.* 62:728, 1949.

230. SZASZ, T. S., KIRSNER, J. B., LEVIN, E., and PALMER, W. L.: "The Role of Hostility in the Pathogenesis of Peptic Ulcer: Theoretical Considerations with the Report of a Case." *Psychosom. Med.* 9:331, 1947.

231. SZONDI, L., and LAX, H.: "Über die Alimentäre Glykämische Reaktion bei Neurasthenie," *Ztschr. f. d. Gesamte Experimentelle Medizin,* 64:274, 1929.

232. TALBOT, N. B., SOBEL, E. H., BURKE, B. S., LINDEMANN, E., and KAUFMAN, S. B.: "Dwarfism in Healthy Children: Its Possible Relation to Emotional, Nutritional and Endocrine Disturbances," *New England J. Med.* 236:783, 1947.

233. TAUBER, E. S., and DANIELS, G. E.: "Further Observations on Androgenic Hormones and Psychic Conflict," *Psychosom. Med.* 11:140, 1949.

234. TAYLOR, H.: "Gastroscopy, Its History, Technique, and Clinical Value with Report on 60 Cases," *Brit. J. Surg.* 24:469, 1937.

235. TOURAINE, G. A., and DRAPER, G.: "The Migrainous Patient," *J. Nerv. & Ment. Dis.* 80:1, 183, 1934.

236. UOTILA, U. U.: "On the Role of the Pituitary Stalk in the Regulation of the Anterior Pituitary, with Special Reference to the Thyrotropic Hormone," *Endocrinology* 25:605, 1939.

237. VAN DER HEIDE, C.: "A Study of Mechanisms in Two Cases of Peptic Ulcer," *Psychosom. Med.* 2:398, 1940.

238. WALLACE, H. L.: "Hyperthyroidism: A Statistical Presentation of its Symptomatology," *Edinburgh M.J.* (N.S.) 38:578, 1931.

239. WEBER, H.: "The Psychological Factor in Migraine," *Brit. J. Med. Psychol.* 12:151, 1932.

240. WEISS, E.: "Cardiospasm: A Psychosomatic Disorder," *Psychosom. Med.* 6:58, 1944.

241. ———: "Psychosomatic Aspects of Hypertension," *J.A.M.A.* 120:1081, 1942.

242. WEISS, E., and ENGLISH, O. S.: *Psychosomatic Medicine.* Second Edition. Philadelphia and London, W. B. Saunders Company, 1949.

243. WEISS, EDOARDO: "Psychoanalyse eines Falles von Nervoesem Asthma," *Internat. Ztschr. f. Psychoanal.* 8:440, 1922.

244. WEISS, S.: "The Interaction between Emotional States and the Cardiovascular System in Health and in Disease," Contributions to the Medical Sciences in Honor of Dr. Emanuel Libman 3:1181, 1932.

245. WEISS, S., and ELLIS, L. B.: "The Quantitative Aspects and Dynamics of the Circulatory Mechanism in Arterial Hypertension," *Am. Heart J.* 5:448, 1930.

246. WESTPHAL, K.: "Untersuchungen zur Frage der nervoesen Entstehung peptischer Ulcera," *Deutsch. Arch. f. Klin. Med.* 114:327, 1914.

247. WHITE, B. V., COBB, S., and JONES, C. M.: *Mucous Colitis.* Psychosom. Med. Monogr. I. Washington, D.C., National Research Council, 1939.

248. WHITE, W. A.: *The Meaning of Disease.* Baltimore, Williams & Wilkins, 1926.

249. WILDER, J.: "Psychological Problems in Hypoglycemia," *Am. J. Digest. Dis.* 10:428, 1943.

250. WILKINS, L., and FLEISCHMANN, W.: "Sexual Infantilism in Females; Causes, Diagnosis and Treatment," *J. Clin. Endocrinol.* 4:306, 1944.

251. WILSON, G. W.: "The Influence of Psychologic Factors upon Gastro-intestinal Disturbances: A Symposium. III. Typical Personality Trends and Conflicts in Cases of Spastic Colitis," *Psychoanalyt. Quart.* 3:558, 1934.

252. WINKELSTEIN, A.: "A New Therapy of Peptic Ulcer," *Am. J. M. Sc.* 185:695, 1933.

253. WITTKOWER, E.: "Studies on the Influence of Emotions on the Functions of the Organs Including Observations in Normals and Neurotics," *J. Ment. Sc.* 81:533, 1935.

254. ———: "Ulcerative Colitis: Personality Studies," *Brit. M.J.* 2:1356, 1938.

255. WOLBERG, L. R.: "Psychosomatic Correlations in Migraine: Report of a Case," *Psychiat. Quart.* 19:60, 1945.

256. WOLFE, T.: "Dynamic Aspects of Cardiovascular Symptomatology," *Am. J. Psychiat.* 91:563, 1934.

257. WOLFF, H. G.: "Personality Features and Reactions of Subjects with Migraine," *Arch. Neurol. & Psychiat.* 37: 895, 1937.

258. WOLFF, H. G., and WOLF, S.: "Studies on a Subject with a Large Gastric Fistula; Changes in the Function of the Stomach in Association with Varying Emotional States," *Tr. A. Am. Physicians* 57:115, 1942.

259. WULFF, M.: "Ueber einen Interessanten Oralen Symptomenkomplex und seine Beziehung zur Sucht," *Internat. Ztschr. f. Psychoanal.* 18:281, 1932.

260. ZWEIG, S.: *Die Heilung durch den Geist (Mental Healers).* Leipzig, Insel-Verlag, 1931.

Index of Names

289

Subject Index

293

Dr. Franz Alexander was born in Hungary and studied medicine and psychiatry at the Universities of Budapest, Cambridge, and Berlin. He came to the United States in 1930 and, in 1932, founded and became the first director of the Chicago Institute for Psychoanalysis. For many years he was Professor of Psychiatry at the University of Illinois. In 1956 he moved to Los Angeles, where he was Director of the Psychiatric and Psychosomatic Research Institute at Mt. Sinai Hospital and Clinical Professor of Psychiatry at the University of Southern California until his recent death. Dr. Alexander is the author of *Fundamentals of Psychoanalysis* and *Psychoanalysis and Psychotherapy*, and was a frequent contributor to the professional journals.

Dr. Therese Benedek was associated with Dr. Alexander for many years at the Chicago Institute for Psychoanalysis. Born in Hungary, she studied at the Universities of Budapest, Possony, and Leipzig before coming to this country. Her books include *Insight and Personality Adjustment* and *Psychosexual Functions in Women*.